Retire to

A BETTER
YOU

How to be *able*
for the rest of your life

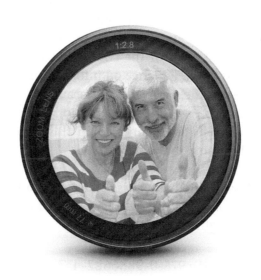

Ed Zinkiewicz

Retire to a Better You: How to Be *Able* for the Rest of Your Life

Copyright © 2013 Retirement-U, Inc.

ISBN (Perfectbound): 978-0-9886622-4-7
ISBN (e-Book): 978-0-9886622-5-4

Cover design and interior layout by Bookcovers.com

Medical Disclaimer

The content in this book and on the related website is for informational purposes only. It is not intended to replace professional medical advice or care from physicians or trained medical professionals. If experiencing symptoms or health problems, seek the advice of your healthcare providers.

Neither Retirement-U, Inc. nor the author provides medical treatment, medical care, or medical advice. No information conveyed by using this book and related website is meant to take the place of your physician or healthcare provider.

You must seek the opinion of a physician for treatment or diagnoses of any medical problem. Do not rely on Retirement-U, Inc. or its products for medical care or medical decision making. Never delay in seeking medical advice or attention because of something you have read in a Retirement-U, Inc. book or on Retirement-U, Inc. website.

IF YOU THINK YOU HAVE A MEDICAL EMERGENCY, CALL YOUR DOCTOR AND 911 IMMEDIATELY!

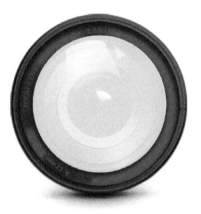

Dedication

I'm grateful for the laughter, the friendship, and yes, Michael, even the pushing that not only kept me coming to water aerobics when I started this journey, but also compelled me to come back. My heartfelt thanks go to many wonderful friends who brought me so much fun while we were enduring together. I will play with any of you again. I have special thanks also for Dale for his joy, encouragement, and an occasional nudge toward the other end of the pool.

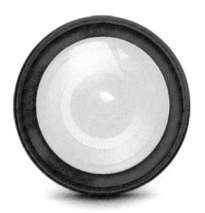

Table of Contents

For You and Footnotes

A website has been created for this book. You can find it at:

www.retireto.info/be-able/bookresources/

In general, the site has two parts:

For You: This part contains additional material you will find helpful in your quest to be able. Most chapters have references at the end that explain material on the site relevant to the chapter. On the website, items are noted by chapter in the For You section.

Footnotes: All of the footnotes from this book are also on the webpage, "bookresources," which is listed above. Some of the footnotes contain web links, which are active there. Just click on them and go directly to the referenced page. In the print version of this book all the web links are shortened. They are limited to their simple home page URL, which makes them easier to type into your browser.

For other resources to help you make your retirement the best of your life, go to retire-to.com.

Bonuses

You may have purchased this book at a brick and mortar or an online bookstore. As a result, you may not have known about the bonuses available to you for purchasing the book.

Don't miss out on these freebies. Just send an email to betteryou@retire-to.com; tell me where you bought the book, if you got this book as a gift and whether you have a paper or electronic version. We'll do the rest.

We'll send you

Let's Get Moving Workbook: The First Four Weeks

Make strides with Erin Pauling's workbook, a guide for those of us who need to start at the beginning. It has a page for each of 28 days with easy-to-follow instructions, tips, and motivational ideas. A professional wellness coach, Erin has a "passion to empower men, women, and children to listen to their hearts and bodies, and enjoy their version of a healthy, balanced life." Check out her website (erinpauling.com).

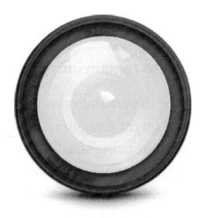

Introduction

I could have cried. I was that happy.

When I read the numbers, they surprised me—and pleased me. I had finally reached a goal that had literally taken years. My waist was 39 inches. It had not been that small for a very long time.

I'll tell you more about the story as the book progresses, but for now, you need to know that I have changed my life. I had to work hard. And from that work, I'm reaching milestones *I never thought I could achieve.*

What took so much work? Eating right and exercising. And you say, "Oh, great. Another lecture on diet and exercise. Yuck!"

You may be asking yourself, "Why bother?" My response is that if you are anything like me, hearing and believing are two very different things. What made a difference for me was to realize finally what was at stake.

Why is all this effort important? Why do I work so hard? I can sum up the answer in a single statement:

I want to remain independent!

I do not want to be dependent on my wife, Crys. I do not want to be dependent on my daughter. I want them to live full and vibrant lives without being shackled with having to care for me—particularly if my efforts might ward off dependence. And I'd rather not be infirm or incapacitated, either.

Continued good health will help me achieve independence. Ongoing commitment to the hard work of eating right and exercising well will help me achieve better health. The loss of inches marked a significant milestone on a road I will continue to travel.

I have a lot of experience with nursing homes.[1] In my frequent visits, I've seen people with a wide range of maladies and abilities. Staff and caregivers must tend the necessary tasks people who are bedridden or in wheelchairs can no longer perform.

On the other hand, I've also spent much time with older adults who have found the retirement facility a headquarters for social contact and meaningful, creative activity. They've given up cooking every meal, mowing the lawn, and keeping up with the house for more time with friends—both old and new—and more activity that is energizing. Taking this step asserts independence.

You don't have to live in a retirement facility to keep active. At the fitness center where I exercise several times a week, I've met others who've inspired me:

---

1   Read about my experiences in the companion book in the "Retire to" series, *Retire to Great Friendships: How to Grow a Network of Fun and Support,* © 2013, Edward J. Zinkiewicz.

- Nola and Thelma, in their seventies, work out five days a week in water aerobics classes.

- Vern and Florence, in their eighties, exercise several days a week. Vern walks laps in the pool, and Florence works out on weight machines and the treadmill.

- Dan and Jack, in their nineties, exercise in the pool several days a week. Both need transportation these days, and Dan has a caregiver who watches from the deck, but both men keep at it.

These folks want to be independent, and they actively and consistently work at that goal.

Not all people who are bedridden or in a wheelchair are there because of their actions. But I don't want to be bedridden or in a wheelchair if I can do things to ensure I'm not.

> *This book is a guide to being able to go, to do, and to maintain independence.*

What about you? Do you want to avoid becoming a burden?

Even if I don't achieve independence that lasts decades, the effort is worth it to me *now*! Why?

I feel better.

I can do more.

My physical indicators have improved—some dramatically.

And, if that's not enough, consider this: I pay less for medications, and my calendar is *not* filled with doctor appointments. Don't those things sound good?

I will never be on TV for what I've achieved—I'm not the "world's biggest loser." But I *am* on track for a happier, longer life because of the course I set five years ago.

Like so many other people, I had expectations of retirement centered on relaxing. I never imagined that retirement would involve so much work! However, you can't reap the reward without the investment—and the investment is paying off.

This book covers several important topics:

- Why adding this work to your life is crucial
- What things you should consider
- Where to go for good advice
- How to get started

What makes this book different from any ad on TV for diet plans or exercise programs? What do *I* have to say that is any better than the advice of "the leading experts"?

The difference is that I've been where you are. I know how to get started. I know how to keep at it. And I know how to tell you about these things. I know what works for many. I know what doesn't. And I'm willing to share.

I don't recommend a single exercise plan, the one-size-fits-all approach. I'll give you many options that will actually sound good to you.

I don't recommend a one-path approach with a single series of steps, either. While I've divided the book into chapters, you drive. You choose the destination. You pick the means. You stay motivated and focused. You lead your advance.

No exercise disk. No motivational videos. No mantras. Just patient, understanding advice about uncomplicated things to do that will help. I talk small steps that mount to big results that will make you proud. I know you can swallow bite-sized options.

To be sure, I will talk about motivation. But I'll talk about motivations that make sense to you and me. You might not want to be an Iron Man or an Iron Woman. That's OK.

But even if you do want that distinction, you need to start somewhere. This book is the place to start.

Let me be your advocate. If you are like me, you need to hear what I have to say. I know you are out there, and I care about what you can achieve.

Although this book is about my success and things I continue to do to make a positive difference in my life, ultimately, it is about who I am and the person I want to be. I am a better person for having done this work. You can be too. I want you to join me.

One last thing: I'm the guy who largely ignored the warning of having had double-bypass surgery. It did not change my life. Yet now, nearly twenty years later, I'm doing a whole raft of things that make a positive difference to my well-being. I'm doing all those things I should have started after surgery, but didn't. Doesn't that raise your curiosity a bit?

The steps I took are ones you can also take. They will take you to a better you. Let me help you start writing *your* book of success.

Your friends and family will notice the difference, as did mine. Let's get going.

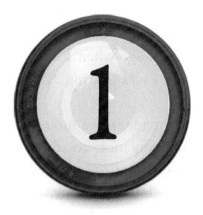

Why I Work So Hard in Retirement

My wake-up call came in two stages.

Stage 1 was the tuxedo. I talked my daughter into a more expensive wedding than it needed to have been because I wanted, once in my life, to wear a tuxedo. Her wedding was a good excuse. I'd never gotten to do that before.

But when I put it on and looked in the mirror, instead of the svelte, dapper, middle-aged father I had imagined, I saw an overweight, apple-shaped advertisement of what eating too much of the "good stuff" can do and, in fact, had done.

Stage 2 happened six years later at the zoo. My wife, Crys, snapped a picture of me with my three-year-old grandson. I was a mess. My belly hung over my belt. My face was bloated. With a white suit, I could have passed for Boss Hogg from *The Dukes of Hazzard*.

At that point in my life, I bet my waist was well over 45 inches. I don't really know because I didn't start keeping records until two years ago when I was at 44 inches. At the time of that zoo trip, I was nearing 210 pounds, an all-time high.[2]

I had that picture made into a mousepad. I gave it to my wife as a promise of many more zoo days with our grandson. Privately, I wondered how many zoo days there could be if I continued to look like I did in that picture.

I hadn't fallen from a place of grace, either. I was never an athlete. I was on the junior high basketball team only because *all* the boys in the class were on the team. I was sedentary. I was a nerds' nerd before nerds were invented. Because I was college-bound and not a high school jock, I thought I had free rein to do as I pleased, which wasn't much.

My mom stepped in at one point. I believe she'd had a discussion with the principal or gym teacher. She hired a high school buddy to "get me in shape." I even think there was some kind of bounty on my head, as guys from the football team came over to invite me to join! They wanted me on the football squad? I don't think so! Very strange.

All this effort was done on the sly, of course. Mom wouldn't or couldn't just tell me I had a problem. She went about fixing it. It didn't occur to me until decades later that the guy I hung out with, the one who invited me to go on bike trips, was there as a fitness coach. We had a good time. And, at the end of the summer, I was able to run a mile without breathing hard. I felt good.

But my physical well-being went down from there. My professional life was spent largely with computers. Throughout

---

2   For my height, I was close to—if not in—Obesity Class II with a body mass index of more than 35.

my career as a computer department manager, programmer, analyst, project manager, data-processing trainer, and consultant, my lifestyle saw no major change. What? I was going to be active by running around the computer? I don't think so!

I did not run.

I did not bike.

I did not swim.

And I was proud that, as in my school-age dream, I worked with my head. I may have worked with my intellect, but I'm here to tell you, I wasn't very intelligent. And I wasn't proud of that picture on the mousepad.

I knew better. I had seen the TV shows, heard the hype about weight, the "apple" shape for men, diet this and diet that. And Crys and I had made some efforts over the years. For example, we started eating better. We ate less beef (encouraged by the fact our daughter gave up beef altogether).

And we exercised—but only sporadically. We joined a fitness center, and I learned how to do the weight machines. If we had a trip coming up, we would walk more "to get in shape to be tourists." Two major trips overseas encouraged a spate of walking to prepare. But nothing seemed to last very long. And we did not do things consistently. None of what we did pushed our limits very far.

So, after that mousepad photo, I decided I needed to start acting in ways that were better for my life. It took three steps to get where I can now write a book and brag. Keep in mind, however, the "steps" are somewhat arbitrary because they were largely accidental.

I did not have a plan. "Better" was the goal at the start. We weren't going for "best in show." And **I did not know how long it would take**, either. So, with that in mind…

Step 1. I had to start somewhere.

I was intentional about this first step. **I had to do something!** But, for me, that was the only certainty. Doing is better than not doing. I preferred to pick something I could do for the long haul, but I didn't have a clue where to start.

I did have a commitment. I didn't want to invest a little and get a little. I wanted to make a difference. It made sense to do something I enjoyed as exercise.

So, I started by buying a bike. My theory was simple—I liked to ride a bike as a kid. Biking in our small town was about the only way we could get around when I was growing up, and even though Mom had slipped money to my friend to take me on bike trips, I had a great time. Besides, nothing else was as appealing to me.

Swimming was out. In college, my swim instructor divided the class into two teams: the rocks and the stones. He didn't think any of us swam very well! And I still swim like a stone. Until recently, my flutter kick took me backward. I'm now working on swimming, but I knew at the outset, swimming was not the place to start.

Running was out as well. I have a long history of lower-back problems. I'm happy to say that I'm definitely making progress in that area. But running was not and probably will not be in the cards because of the fear I have of the continued impact to my back.

I had options with biking. For example, I could use stationary bikes at the gym in the off-season. I could always read while pedaling away, or so I thought.[3] So, bicycle riding was the choice.

---

3   I've since corrected the notion of reading while on the stationary bike. If you are really "going at it," you may not be able to read.

It surprised my wife. Crys frequently goes horseback riding, so my excuse was that I could have something to do while she was out with her horse. To help me get started, I involved my son-in-law. He would ride his bike over to meet me, and we'd go to the nearby greenway to ride the path.

The first few times, I could not do much. No hill was level enough to suit, and each was a strain. I even got off to walk up some hills. And, since I'd purchased the bike in September, I did not have a very long season to get stronger before the snow arrived.

(Yes, I'm a wuss. I don't ride outside in the winter. I didn't say I liked bike riding that much! But I'm glad to report that those hills have smoothed out. Today, I go through those puppies in third gear, but it took a long time to get to that point.)

Later, my wife saw that my biking was not just a passing fancy, so we got her a bike too. While I had had a full spring and summer to practice, she started out with the same problem with those same hills. It wasn't until the following year that we were able to do more riding together.

My improvement program began with a commitment to make a difference doing something physical that I *liked* to do. But because I was still working, that first step of my unplanned program took most of three years.

[Choke!] *Three years? How long is this going to take?*

Keep in mind a couple of things. First, you have this book. I didn't. You know, or soon will know, what to work at. I didn't. You soon will learn through this book that you *can* improve. I didn't know that. I slogged through the meandering, "wind your way across hill and dale and backtrack through the woods" route. You don't have to. So, if you want to improve in less time, go for it—and you will!

Step 2. I had to figure out what to eat.

The second part of the improvement program started when Crys retired two years after I bought my bike. She had her own awakening. When it took her three weeks in bed to recover from the stress and effort to complete a big project at work, she realized that she needed a major change. So, on our way to riding our bikes one day, we talked and agreed that she should stop work.

When she retired, things changed. She committed to eating better and exercising more. So, we began together with regular water aerobics class, more frequent bike riding, and better meals with more dining in instead of out. Unfortunately, because I still worked, I often left the water class after a half-hour to head to the office.

In that phase of our program, we focused on good food. Diet is usually about following a method. We did not need a method. We needed a lifestyle. So, we did not join any brand-name, weight-reducing programs. Instead, we signed up for a twelve-week challenge with a nutrition intern at our wellness center. She provided a log to follow, a few menus, and advice periodically. We did the rest.

And we discussed my retirement.

I was certain of one thing about retirement: I had to retire *to* something and not just *from* something. Although I was very tired of programming computers, I couldn't abandon that post until I claimed a clear reference point out there in the future to head toward. I needed direction. Exercise was growing as one highly likely and significant destination. If I wanted to do anything else in retirement at all, I needed to be *able*.

Step 3. I had to get serious about activity.

During these efforts, Crys began to read. Wellness. Fitness. Heart health. Longevity. Happiness. Every other thing she read pointed to exercise as essential. Some resources spoke of the advantages of exercising. Others pointed out the consequences of not exercising.

So, even though we had made progress toward our goal and definitely felt better, we needed to go further. We took the plunge. I cut my work hours by one-third, and we devoted the extra time to exercise.

Crys and I have committed to exercising vigorously for an hour each day, six days a week. We get up and head for whatever exercise we have planned. We started that practice fourteen months before I retired, and we have continued the regimen since.

We will keep at it too. Why? We'll do it because we have made significant, measurable improvement in our lives![4] And we don't think we're done, either.

So, what about you?

The wake-up call

You need to evaluate two things. First, are you like me? I'm asking whether you've felt the need for a change. And second, have you had a wake-up call?

A wake-up call could be almost anything, and you might have ignored a few. I know I ignored some. I went right on, straight past some things that most people consider serious attention-getters. The double-bypass (nearly twenty years ago) didn't faze me. Say what? How did I ignore that?

---

4   After slimming down from 45 to 39 inches in the waist, losing close to 40 pounds, I'm happy to say while I'm still categorized as "overweight" with a BMI 28.6 (24 will get me to "normal"), I'm no longer on the obese side of the scale! I plan to be done with obese forever!

Apparently, it was easy. Inertia is a powerful thing. I just kept on keeping on. After the bypass, I did not change my lifestyle significantly. Oh, I joined the wellness center and worked out a little. But I did not make the *big* change until I had a grandson.

I'm sorry to say, I didn't heed my wife, either. She knew exercise was important. She was encouraging. She saw the mess I was in and wanted better for me. And although I heard and was sympathetic, her concern for me did not result in change. I'm not proud of that. I can say the same thing about my daughter. Her concern for my well-being did not move me to improve.

My wake-up call was really a series of things:

Wife's concern
+ Bypass surgery
+ Daughter's concern
+ Grandson
= **Wake up!**

How about you? Had any wake-up calls lately? I encourage you to look. Have you ignored some warnings? More than one? Are they piling up?

Imagine the wake-up call as an avalanche. An avalanche starts as a snowfall. Over time, snow piles up on a ledge—a ledge perched above your head. You notice the change up there in an offhand, distant way and say to yourself, "My, isn't the snow pretty." Time passes. Snow accumulates. The frozen layers compress and deepen. You can't or won't move out of the way. One fine, clear crisp winter day, you hear a sharp report! A deep rumble starts under your feet. Everything crashes down. When you awake, you realize that whatever happened has moved you in a new direction.

Are you paying attention? Is the snow becoming denser above your head? Do you remember the concerns of your loved ones? Do you hear—at last—the appealing tone in your doctor's latest report? Have you read yet another article that heaps on a layer of reasons you need a change?

Dense as I am, the message eventually got through. So, what do *you* find when you look back over the years?

Are you ready to listen and to *act*? Your buying this book is a good sign. You're taking a positive step. You not only know you need to do something, but also you are willing to put your money where your mouth is. Good for you.

If you want a refresher on why you should take serious action, consider the following:

- Retirees fear infirmity later in life because their lack of independence will not only burden them but also their family. Do you want to be a burden to your family?
- If you are not a burden to your family, your family can live more fully.
- If you choose your exercise efforts wisely, you can get back in touch with something adults often lose—a sense of play. Do you remember how fun it was to play?
- Feeling better and being able to do more means you can enjoy life more. You are happier. You laugh more. You have more fun. Wouldn't fun be… fun?
- If you can do more and feel better, you are better able to help others. I thought that was important. Do you think so too?
- If you don't get up and go, you may find that your get-up-and-go got up and went. Use it or lose it!

One last note about wake-up calls. You can create your own "avalanche" to get yourself going. You don't have to wait for circumstances and consequences to crowd you. Do some informal interviews. Ask your family members some questions:

- Are they worried about you?
- What concerns do they have about caring for you long term?
- If long-term care for you were off the radar for your family, how would they choose to live? What hopes do they have? How might you help them?
- What's fun for you? How might you play more? Think about things you can do as a family if you are physically able. Start planning to do them. Be sure to include steps that will mean you're well enough to enjoy life.
- How might you serve? In what ways could you help others—if you were able?

At one point, I asked my wife for a list. I asked her for ten reasons I needed to get stronger. I tacked it up so I could see it as a reminder.

Create a second list and do similar interviews with friends and colleagues about their hopes and what they are doing for themselves. I didn't know that the data-processing manager at work was using a kettle ball. I asked questions and added another possible activity to my list. How many friends do you have? Get started with those conversations!

Above all, don't wait for a wake-up call. Jump in anyway. The first steps don't hurt. I promise. Read the next chapter, and see where it takes you.

A word about expense

We all know the phrase "put your money where your mouth is." If you want to "walk the talk," you will make a financial commitment. You have to "pay your dues." Enough clichés?

OK, I'll quit. Here is the point: You have to spend some money. How much? That depends.

Things to consider:

1. Some activities do not have heavy start-up costs, but others might tax your budget. Swimming, for example. Unless you have access to a free pool, finding a place to swim will likely mean a monthly investment in a Y or other gym membership.

2. Running is less expensive. You don't have to rent a running track (that is, join a gym or fitness center) unless the winter where you live makes outdoor activity unwise. You may need cool-weather clothing. You will definitely need good shoes, and you will need to replace them even when the tops still look good. (You need to pay attention to the wear on the bottom. That's what matters.) In other words, expense varies with the activity you choose.

3. Expense also varies with your level of involvement. My wife and I do not compete in bicycle races, nor do we travel across the state or country to find cycling events. But both are options, and the cost would go up with each trip taken.

4. Our friend Emma goes around the country to compete in Senior Olympic swimming events (successfully, we're proud to say, even though we can't take any credit). She doesn't have heavy-duty expense because of her choice of activity, but her expenses are higher than those of other swimmers who do not travel to compete.

5. You are not buying new toys—you are buying "lifesaving" equipment. The expense we're talking about is an investment in yourself. Don't skimp on gear. Good gear can protect your body; bad gear can tear up your hard-earned advances.

6. Any equipment you purchase now will almost certainly cost less than medical costs you would incur because of not exercising.

7. Expenses might be offset by insurance or written off on taxes if it is part of a prescribed medical care plan. Talk to your doctor and tax person.

8. Exercise gear changes rapidly, which means you can count on regular improvements in the gear that will make performance better. Consequently, you may want to purchase gear that matches your performance now and later buy better gear to match your improved performance.

9. You may also need help along the way. Consultant advice is available through these sources, which I've listed generally in order of expense:

   - A store
   - A club
   - A fitness center or exercise facility
   - A class
   - Personal attention

If you have questions, it costs less to ask the clerk in the red shirt at the store than it does to work with a personal trainer. The level of advice given (or even the level of ability to give good advice) is also listed here lowest to highest. A store clerk is more focused on sales and less knowledgeable and skilled than a personal trainer is—usually.

So, now you are awake. Right? Maybe you've heard your wake-up call. Maybe not. But where do you begin?

In Chapter 2, we help you get started. We emphasize finding something you *like* to do rather than asking you to jump into the deep end. We don't advocate going overboard;

we encourage a natural progression of effort that counts on your learning to pay attention to *your* body. We offer ideas to help you get going and keep going.

In Chapter 3, we help you ramp up the level of activity in your life. We introduce monitoring results—and cool tools for keeping track. We talk about goals that can change how you feel about more activity—and, more important, improve what you *can* do.

Finally, in Chapter 4, we turn attention to what you eat. We give you commonsense, reasonable steps that can help you transform your daily food choices into healthier ones.

A better you won't just happen. But step-by-step, you can be more *able* for the rest of your life.

For You

Just to help you get going on the right track, I've included a "wake-up" interview sheet for you on a special website built exclusively for those who've purchased this book:

www.retireto.info/be-able/bookresources/

And, just so you get the picture, I'll include some of my photos—the non-svelte proud father at his daughter's wedding, the much chubbier proud grandfather a few years later, and a more recent, improved (and proud) me. The pictures give you a starting reference. Look at the site and see.

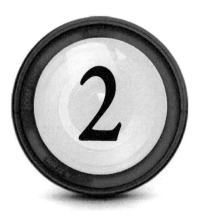

Get Started[5]

A journey of a thousand miles begins with a single step.
–Lao-tzu (Chinese philosopher 604–531 B.C.)

You only have one question to answer: What do you like to do?

Hold on—not so fast! Before you embark on a new program, you really *need* to talk to your doctor. But before you can do that, you need to know what to talk about. So, let's start by considering options. After you and your doctor agree on a starting place, *then* you begin.

---

5 Time for the disclaimer: I'm not a doctor. I'm not a nutritionist. I don't train people for athletic events. I'm a nerd. I know this: What I've done works for me. But I took proper precautions by talking with my doctor and seeking the advice of people who should know about next steps. So, before you continue to read, check out the disclaimer at the beginning of this book. I can't guarantee your success. But I do believe what has worked for me is a good recipe for many. Ultimately, you have to decide your course of action and be responsible for its consequences, whether known or unintended.

The bottom line is that you need to start somewhere. Inactivity is bad. Activity gives you energy. Your age is just a number and no predictor for how vital you are.

So, you have two things to do right now:

1. Consider the options.
2. Put pedal to the metal.

Consider the options.

What do you like?

> *Don't stop now!*
>
> Activity is good. On the other hand, inactivity will help prove the adage:
>
> *When you're 20, you're hot.*
> *When you're 40, you're not.*
> *When you're 60, you're shot.*
>
> Yikes! Don't tell my wife. I keep telling her she's hot. And though she's a few years past 20, she's hot because she keeps on going.

I suggest starting with what you like because it's best to be on a road you want to travel. Remember, I started with biking because I liked it. It turned out that to get better at biking, I needed to improve overall muscle tone. So, I moved to doing floor exercises under a trainer's guidance for a while. Now, floor work is part of my weekly schedule.

Because of the floor work, the range of biking venues open to me has improved. I can do the hilly rides now. I can ride longer. I enjoy bikes even more! I'm still not where I can brag about how many dozens of miles I ride at a stretch. But I think that's partly because biking is not *the* central activity anymore. I have a larger range now that includes water aerobics, tai chi, hiking, floor work, and walking—both inside on the treadmill and track and outside in the sunshine.

I'm happy to say that because of these, I am able to play more with my grandson. Together, we like to creek walk, play disc golf, hike, and bike.

Ideally, then, you want to think of a big list. What about…

- Walking
- Swimming
- Water aerobics
- Hiking
- Biking
- Running
- Dancing or Zumba
- Fitness machines (the elliptical, The StairMaster, and so forth)
- Kayaking
- Canoeing
- Snorkeling
- Skating (on ice or road)
- Skiing (and variations)
- Yoga
- Pilates
- Floor or step aerobics
- Kick boxing
- Kettle ball

And the list can go on and on.

If you have a clear-cut idea of where to start, you can move to the "Put pedal to the metal" section of this chapter. If you need some help thinking about how to begin, here are some suggestions:

What are your friends doing?

You stay active to help yourself, but you can also enjoy good company while you do it. One thing that keeps Crys and me going to water aerobics each week is the friends we have there.

We've gotten to know folks. We laugh together. Exercise has added a social component. It's much more fun that way.

Do folks who like this activity mingle?

When you begin to explore options, check out other social opportunities too. The store where we bought our bikes offers monthly riding activities. A quick Internet search will give you a variety of interest groups that focus on one or more activities on your list.

For example, a search for "running clubs" in my area produced several pages of options and opportunities. Our Nashville Striders hosts organized runs, parties, networking and volunteer opportunities; puts out a monthly newsletter; and gives discounts on merchandise. More ways to stay active! You'll no doubt find similar clubs or organizations in your area too.

Check out the interest groups for your chosen pursuit. You will likely find beginner activities, training events, coaching, and advice on equipment. A website called Meetup might just be the ticket for finding what you want to do and great people with whom to do it near you.

You don't have to make a lifetime commitment. Use the opportunity to see what an activity is about before you decide it is for you. And even if you take up the activity, you don't have to stay with the group.

What's in all those scrapbooks from long ago?

Think about what you enjoyed doing when you were younger. Did you hike as a kid with your family or Scout troop? Run track in high school? Star on the college swim team? Your history may provide a clue to how to stay active now that you've retired. Maybe you didn't do any of those things, but wished you could.

Well, here is good news: Now, you have the time!

Your list probably has more things on it than you can do on a daily basis. The next step, then, is to prioritize. Consider ranking them according to

- Level of aerobic activity
- Level of strength building
- Expense
- Availability of training
- Availability of social contact
- How long it takes to get there
- Year-round availability

What can you no longer do?

The other day, I watched a lean and trim 70-year-old-plus man running the elliptical. I take that back. He wasn't just running—he was sprinting for all he was worth. I've not seen that much effort put into that machine very often. He came off the machine soaked in sweat. I was worn out just watching.

When we talked, he called himself a runner. But he said he was a runner at heart only, because due to arthritis, his feet could no longer take the impact. Arthritis did not stop him, though. He still exercises.

So, where are you? Making substitutions is common. Our friend Cheryl had to stop running, so she chose swimming because it's easier on the body, and she knew she could do it for the rest of her life.

Inability to no longer do an activity is not a "get out of jail free" card. It just means you have to be more selective.

Check with your doctor.

This bears repeating: Don't start anything new without checking with your doctor about exercise.

Take your list of possible activities when you go, because it is an important starting point for discussion. You want him or her to evaluate the aerobic and strength-building activities. It may turn out that activity X is far more likely to be strength building for you than activity Y. This input about the relative result of activities may influence your choice.

The list also gives your doctor a place to start the discussion of your physical ability to meet the challenge. Don't be surprised if your doctor asks to run tests. (In fact, many wellness centers require new members to provide a doctor's OK before exercise can begin.)

It's also a good idea to have options because your doctor may want you to reconsider some of your choices. He or she may suggest you begin with something less (or more) strenuous. You might have some physical condition that prohibits activity in one area or another. Or he or she might question some choices because of the risk of injury. Running puts more pressure on joints than swimming or biking, for example. Some activities such as tennis involve joint and tendon impact as well. Your doctor can let you know.

Passing the test

When I joined the wellness center affiliated with a local hospital, I was required to have an OK from my doctor before I could take a class.

My doctor had me do a stress test. Because I'd already had a bypass operation and was not in the best shape (to be generous about it), the test was probably a very good idea.

But the experience took me back to the good old days when we had to have a doctor's form to start school!

Do not skip this step:
Check with your doctor before you begin.

Put pedal to the metal.

Are you a bit curious about how well an exercise program will work for you? Or are you anxious or nervous—afraid you will fail?

What are you worried about?

Can I do it? The human body is a wonderful instrument. In general, if you do the things you need to do to improve, your body will support the effort. It will rise to meet the challenge. The human body is built for more physical activity than most of us can achieve sitting

> **You can only fail if you don't try.**

at a desk or driving from place to place. So, unless you push yourself recklessly, you don't have to worry whether your body will keep up.

Can I afford it? Generally, you can justify the expense of equipment or gym membership by the health benefits you gain. As we've said, the cost of good gear trumps medical healthcare costs you are likely to incur if you do not exercise. And don't skimp on safety equipment if you choose an activity that calls for it. I've seen the results of brain injuries, so I always wear a helmet riding a bicycle. Check with a local store that specializes in equipment for your activity. You can easily find out what gear is recommended because they probably sell it.

Will I be embarrassed because I'm out of shape? You might worry about what you look like to others at the gym. Remember in the movie *Predator* when Arnold Schwarzenegger finally pulls the mask off the alien enemy? He says, "You are one ugly..." (expletive intentionally deleted).

Guess what? Nobody at the gym pulled off my mask. All the members of my highly trained, exquisitely sculpted team at water aerobics are examples of peak human performance, just as I am (cough, cough). And so, I assume they are equally interested in keeping that mask on. Thank you very much.

Translation: Folks are too busy dealing with their own appearance to worry about yours.

Once you get the gear and safety equipment, appearance and expense, and the anxiety or nervousness out of the way, the first step of your exercise plan is very simple—just show up!

Plan what you do based on a little self-assessment. If you intend to swim laps, for example, think about how long it's been since you swam. If you have not done it in a while, you might want to try it by yourself before you commit to a lap class. If the basics are too far behind, you can schedule work with a trainer for a short time. If the basics are still in place, then you still may want to work on your own for a bit, building up some endurance, before committing to a lap class.

On the other hand, if you get the old (good) form back in a week, have at it. Schedule a regular time, and go for it. Or join a lap class to have the advantages of a trainer who can help you focus on fundamentals and essentials and the camaraderie of others who are also swimming for their health. However you choose to begin, the key is *to begin!* Then keep at it—you will improve.

The same advice applies to nearly any activity:

> Assess your current skill level.
> Plan your initial activity around your current level.

Start at a comfortable level. Then, keep at it. Chris Crowley, the author of *Younger Next Year*, offers this bit of encouragement:

Don't feel like an idiot if you can barely stay on the treadmill for fifteen minutes at low speed the first day.... It is not struggling on the first day or the thirtieth or sixtieth that's going to work. It's showing up every day and doing something.[6]

Don't overextend yourself. You don't train to run the marathon by running 26 miles your first time. Everything has a starting point. You have to live with yours. You can improve. You don't want to take six weeks off at the beginning of your exercise program to recover from whatever it was that you did on the first day!

The opposite is true as well. You don't want to start at a low level and stay there. You want to improve. Don't overextend, but don't forget to extend, either.

How much is enough?

When I began to get serious about exercise, as I chronicled earlier, it took two months for me to get into bike riding and a couple of years before it became a leisure activity. It took quite a while to get into exercising in the pool as well. When I started, all I did was walk—forward, backward, and sideways. I measured progress with the number of laps, which was embarrassingly low to start.

After a while, I joined my wife in a moderately paced water exercise class for two days a week. The instructor was Barb, and she made the class fun and challenged us with water activities we'd not tried before. Can you sit on a foam noodle and pedal your way to the deep end? You should have seen us the first time. Barb emphasized stretching, flexibility, and balance exercises.

---

6   Christopher Crowley, Henry S. Lodge, *Younger Next Year: Live Strong, Fit, and Sexy—Until You're 80 and Beyond,* © 2004, 2005, p. 84.

We got a new instructor, Stephen, for the three-day-a-week water aerobics class. Stephen specialized in Ironman Triathlon coaching; needless to say, our class became more strenuous. It also became fun because Stephen also had us playing with beach balls.

Then Michael came. It is difficult to describe Michael. He was sort of a cross between drill sergeant and teddy bear. When he started with us, we weren't sure what we'd gotten into. "Down to the deep end. Get your weights. Run back. No, I said run!" And when we'd gotten back to the shallow end, it was, "Drop those weights. Swim back to the deep end." Oops.

Did I mention that I don't swim well? Hmm. I hung in there. My wife hung in there. Michael was probably the best thing that happened to the class—and to me. We all got stronger. I can swim now—first time since college. I have more endurance and flexibility too. And Crys, now in a regular lap class, swims laps two times a week for an hour both days.

She and I were very happy with Stephen because we got stronger. We were delighted with Michael. We learned that we could push ourselves. Michael never made us do more than we could as individuals and often split the class so he could tailor activities to different groups.

He had an uncanny knack for spotting slackers. But he also watched like a hawk to be sure that we were not in danger, and he was careful to plan activities that compensated for recent strains or that helped prepare for coming events. For example, several months before knee surgeries, Michael helped two of our members work on strength building to bolster their recovery after surgery. These women both claimed shorter recovery times than others who had the same surgeries at the same time. That's how Michael showed us his teddy bear side.

This story chronicles some lessons I learned:

First, I did not start water activity at a high level. I did what I could do.

Second, I kept at it. This whole pool story took a couple of years.

Third, I learned to push myself while also paying attention to my body. I grew with continued effort.

You can follow the same course. But you have to get in the pool, so to speak, to get started.

What if you don't like it?

However, you don't have to stay in the pool. Consider an initial foray into any activity as an experiment. What happens if you don't like it? You have a wealth of other options.

As much as I want you to dive into exercise with a commitment to continue, finding something you like to do is important. Your interest in the activity is what will get you started and keep you going. Don't give up. Change up if you have to or if you want to. The goal is to develop the yearning to keep exercising.

If bicycling is your first choice, many cities provide bicycles and gear for public use. Find a bike loan location, get on, ride around, and take the bike back. Or maybe you have a friend with a bike who will let you try it. Borrowed equipment might not be the ideal solution, but this way, at least you can learn whether bicycle riding is as much fun as you remember.

Or start with a good secondhand bike. If you find the terrain in your area is too challenging or you really don't like riding, you can resell the equipment and start over. If you find that biking has become a component of the new-you lifestyle, you can invest in better equipment.

Similarly, you might commit to an eight-week membership at the gym to join the step-aerobics class (water aerobics class, tai chi class, yoga class, martial arts class, Zumba class). If you like the class and the other amenities the facility offers, you can extend the membership.

On the other hand, you might want to try another gym and another class for the next six or eight weeks. You might find that you appreciate the instructor from one place better than another or one set of facilities over another. You might need more intensity or less. With short-term memberships, you can experiment.

Crys and I are fortunate that our Medicare provider gives us complimentary membership to *Silver Sneakers*,[7] a nationwide fitness program for older adults. This means we can participate in any YMCA in the area, and we have tried several. Now, we have choices.

Having a variety of alternatives is important. Choice of exercise venues and types

- Keeps interest up.
- Provides rainy-day alternatives.
- Keeps options open while traveling. (We feel comfortable picking from a short list of things available at a strange place because we've done many of them.)
- Exercises different muscle groups.
- Allows a varied pace (aerobics one day, flexibility training the next).

7 You can find details of Silver Sneakers at www.silversneakers.com. This site will tell you which health plans support the program, give directions to facilities, and provide more information.

When things go bump

You know the rule about getting back on the horse after a fall, right? Try as we might, being as careful as we can while doing our best, we might hurt ourselves. Goodness, I bent over to flush the toilet some months back, and my back went into spasms. What is up with that? It did not happen while exercising!

For me, the sad news is clear—my back is my most vulnerable part. I've sent muscles into spasm from working too hard and from working too little. I've bent over to grab my gym bag, lifted the tailgate on the car, and picked up a suitcase with similar results. The pain is instantaneous and sometimes extreme. The result has laid me low for days or weeks.

You, too, will sprain something. You will have sore muscles. You can also be sick. Allergies have on occasion slowed me to a point that heavy exercise is impossible. Such illnesses or injuries often have nothing to do with my exercise program.

It doesn't matter what slowed you or how it happened. The question is, What do you do about it?

Recovery for me follows a standard routine. I slow down, but I keep moving. I'm careful, and I build back up

Pay attention to your body

You need to extend yourself. But a little push goes a long way. When you exercise, build in a second step. Here are some examples:

If you try something new one day, do something familiar the next. The same is true of intensity. If you do something very intense one day, make a different choice for the next day. I don't do floor work two days in a row. I always break it up with some kind of water aerobics.

If you have a new ache today, be sure to learn what stretch will help relieve the discomfort.

If you have pain (worse than "aches"), evaluate. You can stop what you're doing and come back to it another day or simply do it more gently. Pay attention to your body. On the other hand, if you have pain several times in a row, something may be wrong. Seek help.

gradually to the level I had before the incident. I have a "slow and gentle" water aerobics class that helps keep me going. The bottom line is simple—don't let illness or injury derail your program.

You will avoid some strains and sprains by warming up before you start exercising. Adding a slow-down period and stretching at the end will help you avoid soreness. If you are in a class, chances are the instructor will build in these elements. Pay attention. You want to learn *how* so you can repeat the pattern on your own, if need be. Don't skip the warm-ups at the beginning and stretching at the end.

My doctor friend Richard also advises that "joint replacement puts limits on what exercise can be done but is not a license to stop; exercise should be continued." I agree and can cite examples of people who have pulled themselves through replacement surgery and continued. Richard is one. Surgery can be a setback. It might change or limit what you do, but the goal remains. Keep moving.

A distinction

Before we finish this chapter, let's make a distinction. There is exercise, and there are leisure activities. To bring them together, remember this: Exercise gives you the strength, flexibility, and stamina to do the leisure activities (without hurting yourself).

What are leisure activities? They may include some things folks want to do more of when they retire. Leisure activities include things such as golf and tennis and horseback riding.

I know some of you will be pained by this distinction, which is why I left this discussion to the end of the chapter. I know you looked forward to playing more golf in your retirement and felt good about "getting more exercise" in the process. Go ahead and play golf. You will burn calories and build strength for a specific, repetitive set of motions. You will get out in the sun. You will be with friends. But you will not be building endurance, or overall strength, or getting an aerobic workout. On the other hand, if you forgo the golf cart and walk the entire nine or eighteen holes, you will have exercised. Walking is good for you in general.

To be fair, while getting better, you may find some things you used to call exercise may transform into leisure activities. Riding my bike on the greenway is not the challenge for me it once was, for example. As you become fit, some things you did at first for exercise now become the "fun" things, the extra things. Feeling better helps you enjoy more active pursuits.

How do you know the difference between leisure activities and activities that improve your health? You have to learn to measure levels of activity. You have to learn to evaluate what is happening as it is happening. You need to involve your doctor on your journey toward fitness, not just at launch time when you start. In short, you need to get serious about exercise.

For You

To help you get started with a fun exercise choice, I've included a small workbook on a special website exclusively for those who've purchased this book:

www.retireto.info/be-able/bookresources/

The workbook will help you find and evaluate options.

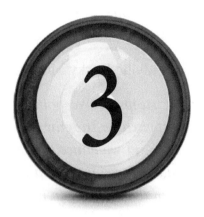

Get Serious

What do you mean by "serious"?

In about Year 3 of our migration toward fitness, my wife, Crys, and I read *Younger Next Year*, a book by Chris Crowley (with coauthor Henry S. Lodge, MD), which encourages us Baby Boomers (and older) to stay fit and healthy. Chris' transformation from high-powered lawyer to ski bum to fitness guru really captured my interest. One story about skiing in powder snow was motivating:

> *That's one of the dirty little secrets about skiing that the instructors and ski magazines never mention. Skiing is a strength sport. Aerobics and strength. The stronger and fitter you are, the more fun you have…. There's technique*

and there's balance. But, time and again, strength and fitness are what make it possible. Especially in powder.[8]

Chris described an idyllic Rocky Mountain scene:

We were in the steeps…. We pointed our skis straight down the steepest pitch…. The gravity pulled us down, the snow held us up. And we danced in between. [We] were flying, side by side. We grinned, and we whooped. All the way down. Down the steep, open hill, down through the huge trees in The Glades. Up and across to the Ridge of Bell and into the steeps again.

He and his friend Lois laughed, played, and ran the run repeatedly. With small breaks and a light lunch, they found themselves "cooked" after five hours. Yet, they still managed to giggle and boast and commend each other. "We thought we were wonderful."

Do you hear the joy in his voice? Do you see the vistas laid out for him and his skiing partner? Can you imagine the open sky, white powder snow, swatches of evergreen, the purity of the air, and the chill against your face? It sounds magnificent. Chris made this ski trip when he was 70.

Yikes! I don't ski, so I don't have a clue about what it takes to do what he did. I understand why he needed that three-hour nap after. I could probably handle the nap part, but I'm sure I couldn't do what he did for five hours straight. Chris was aerobically fit. He was strong. He had endurance. He had flexibility and mobility.

Chris' journey to fitness involved steady improvement in physical ability with consistent work. I doubt I'll be skiing at 70, but as I read this story, I sat up straight and started paying

8 *Younger Next Year, Live Strong, Fit, and Sexy—Until You're 80 and Beyond,* by Chris Crowley and Henry S. Lodge, M.D. Copyright " 2007 by Chris Crowley and Henry S. Lodge. Published by Workman Publishing Company.

attention. What a wonderful conclusion—to feel that good after that much exertion! I wanted to know more. I wanted to do more. I wanted to feel that good. I wanted to be *able* to do what I love too!

Once I had read Chris' story, I began to see articles about accomplishments of people my age. It was like buying a new car—as soon as you get yours, you begin to notice how many of the same cars are traveling the roads with you.

Here's another: Nadine Rihani of Nashville is 73 and ran her eleventh marathon in 2012. She began to run at 61. In a newspaper article about her accomplishment, Nadine says:

> *"Sometimes I don't even tell people I do marathons, because they look at me differently. A lot of my friends like to play bridge."*[9]

Go, Nadine! I want you to tell me more. I want Chris Crowley to tell me more. I want all these heroes to keep proclaiming that there is life after retirement. Retirees can do these wonderful physical feats. Their stories keep me going and doing what I do to stay fit.

My wife, Crys, and I began our journey into this level of activity by riding bicycles. That was only the beginning. Our path has broadened and evolved. But the transformation began with the simple rule stated in Chris Crowley's book:

> *Exercise six days a week for the rest of your life.*

No negotiation. No excuses. Get out and do it.

My wife's cousin, Carolyn Petty (about the same age as we are), adds another motivator; she posted on Facebook:

> *I can stretch and work out or I can hurt. I know this. I've known it for twenty years. Saturday I skipped it as*

---

9 "Age Is No Excuse," by Tony Gonzalez, *The Tennessean*.

I attempted to make every minute count, working on several projects. Sunday: nearly pain free. Yesterday: Tin Woodsman needing oil can. Today: wall-to-wall pain. Lesson: I can stretch and work out or I can hurt. My choice.

Here's what you need to remember when you set out to follow this rule, which will help keep the hurt at bay:

- Emphasize exercise
- Find a partner
- Measure results
- Track results

Emphasize exercise.

In Chapter 2 of this book, we talked about treating exercise as play. When I started riding a bicycle again, I wanted something to do that I could enjoy so I would keep doing it.

Now, it is time to transition. How do we get more fit so the play will be more fun? How do we get to where we can ski for five hours straight, as Chris Crowley described, or perform any activity we choose with that level of intensity, exhilaration, and enjoyment?

Can I ski or achieve that level of activity for five hours straight? Not yet. But I do feel better because I've moved in that direction. I can do much more today than I could last year.

Exercise seems to encourage exercise. That might sound foreign. To me—the original and highly advanced couch potato—those words coming out of my mouth sound unbelievable. But the statement is true. I *feel* like doing more because I *can* do more.

How did I get there? Crys and I developed a formula that helps keep us on track:

- Treat exercise as a job.
- Exercise on a fixed schedule.
- Join a gym.
- Get a buddy.
- Take a class.
- Have fun.

Treat exercise as a job.

I mentioned our friends Vern and Florence earlier in this book. We met them at our wellness center several years ago. They exercise most days of the week. "We treat it like a job," said Vern.

Time to get up and go to work. Vern's attitude just makes sense. After all, work is not a problem. You and I know how to do that. By the time people retire, they have spent decades getting up and out for work. Every day. Every week. What's the problem? We worked most days of our lives.

At the time we heard this, Crys and I were still working. So, while the hint from Vern and Florence sounded good, Crys found it nearly impossible to practice. Frequently, yes. Regularly, no. But because I was a "consultant" with flexible hours, I started to go to the pool regularly. I'd head off to the pool and leave from there to go to the current job site. I didn't always stay long. I didn't improve much. But I did go.

When Crys retired, scheduled exercise helped solve another pressing concern—what do I do all day? In that light, regular exercise seemed an easy thing to do. Exercise first; then, move on to the rest of the day.

Currently, in our week, you will find us in a strenuous water aerobics class Monday, Wednesday, and Friday. Tuesday is Crys' riding day. She volunteers with *Saddle Up!*, a therapeutic riding program for children with disabilities. My Tuesday exercise is usually tai chi. I sometimes add another water class or do floor work.

Thursday finds Crys back in the pool for a lap class, and it's my day to do cross training with weights and walking or to attend another water aerobics class across town. Saturday, we're on our bikes or at another water aerobics class or doing our workout in the pool. We've even been known to participate in a water spin class occasionally. Yep! Bikes in the pool!

Crys and I are equal opportunity water-class folks. We go where the classes are challenging. Because of our membership in *Silver Sneakers,*[10] we can participate in any Y in the area, and we have tried several in Nashville.

Variety is an important part of the routine Crys and I have established. It changes things up, keeps interest high, and gives us some flexibility. When the lightning storm comes to town, we don't have to worry about the pool being closed; we can do floor work or join a step aerobics class for the day.

Please recognize there are no five-hour runs down powdery slopes in this routine. Crys and I are not in that league. If you read Chris Crowley's *Younger Next Year*, you will find that the author's hard work in the gym on a regular schedule makes the extraordinary stories possible.

Thanks to our commitment to exercise six days a week, my wife and I have stories to tell as well. They just are not as extreme. We were both able to take our bikes on vacation and do what was, for us, a much longer bike trip. And Crys is happy to report that because of the lap swimming she does regularly, she can now swim longer and stronger than before.

---

10 We mentioned this earlier, but in case you missed it, you can find details of Silver Sneakers at www.silversneakers.com. This site will answer your questions, tell you which health plans support the program, and give directions to facilities.

If Chris Crowley and Dr. Lodge have it right, next year, Crys and I will be able to do even more!

Exercise on a fixed schedule.

There is no louder death-knell to an exercise program than the "I'll catch that as I can" approach. After all, that's exactly how I avoided regular exercise for decades!

We do our exercise as the first activity of the day. Generally, that makes our exercise program even more like a job. On the other hand, if you work now and exercise regularly, your challenge in retirement may simply be to establish a new "normal." What fits into your retirement schedule?

A regular exercise regimen on a fixed schedule minimizes decisions. It's 8 A.M? Good. Time to go to class. None of the "Do I have time to go to class today?" Or worse, "Do I want to go to class today?" Eight in the morning means it is time. So, go.

A regular program is also easy to schedule around. "Sorry, can't meet at 9 A.M. I have an appointment with my *(name your favorite exercise here).*"

My wife and I conduct a workshop called *The New 3R's of Retirement.*[11] One of my favorite activities in that workshop is to learn what people think they will miss when they leave work (or what they have already missed). A common answer to the question is structure—the act of getting up and going to work, day in, day out, at the same time.

It seems that some people have a hard time getting up in the morning. Our friend Marcia claims she'd never get out of her jammies if there weren't a real "I have to be there" schedule in hand. If you are one of those folks who would miss structure, setting a standard time for exercise may get you out of a jam (pun intended).

---

11 You can check out this course and other resources at Retirement-U.com.

Join a gym.

If money is involved somehow, exercising seems more important. My wife and I cannot afford to waste limited resources. So, having paid, we go.

On the other hand, the expense may be a worry if there is little return. I remember our discussion six years ago about whether to continue our membership at the local wellness center because we felt we weren't getting our money's worth. You have to walk a fine line. There needs to be some compelling activity to justify the expense, even as the expense may motivate activity. It really is a chicken-and-egg deal.

We would not think of canceling our membership now. We wonder how they keep the volume of towels we use clean for what we pay every month! But we have no question on our end whether to pay. We really use the facility. Consider that, with our membership, we have year-round access to

- A pool
- A track
- Weight machines and free weights
- Instructors and advisors
- Classes
- Seasonal challenges (keep weight off through holidays)
- A hot tub
- A steam room
- A massage therapist
- And people glad to see us!

The built-in variety the center offers is enough to keep us, if not pleasantly, then strenuously occupied, which is more than I can say for doing exercise at our house and in our neighborhood. I'll never need cold-weather gear at the gym to use the track, but I certainly would if I chose to walk outdoors year-round.

If you are someone who needs structure in your life, having a gym membership is a plus. It is easier to go to work when there is a place to go. The same is true for exercise.

Over your lifetime, the activities you choose may change. My wife and I spend a lot of time in the pool now, but we started our exercise program on bicycles. Although we puchased the gym membership so we could have access to a pool, we both walk the track and do a group floor exercise class. I use the weight machines, as well.

Consider convenience. You do not want to waste exercise time in travel. Finding parking might be difficult at some places. Use the time it takes from your front door to the locker as the basic unit of comparison.

Get a buddy.

You won't blow off a buddy! Right? So, when it comes time to get to the gym, head for the pool, get on the bike, put the mittens on, or toss the ice skates over your shoulder, having a friend at your destination will help make exercise more palatable.

A lot of stuff you do in exercise, you do alone. But having a buddy who does the same stuff right by your side makes it a little more inviting. After all, parallel play is the first kind we learn. We've likely been practicing it for many years.

You can even spot for each other. I tell Crys to roll on her side into that backstroke! She tells me not to just stand there yakking at her, but *swim*!

Maybe you can jog with a friend, bike with a group, swim on a team, or practice with a coach. There are dozens of ways to find a buddy.

Take a class.

Another buddy system that works for us is a class. Crys and I have been in the same water aerobics class for several years. We've had various instructors during that time. The current one pushes us, offers a lot of variety, pays attention to what we can do, and helps us with advice and encouragement. Crys and I (and I believe the rest of the class) have become stronger during this instructor's tenure.

We've learned more about what we're doing and why, as well. Our instructor will often report, "Today, we emphasized working on that muscle group" or "This stretch is for such-and-so muscle group."

But the benefits of participating in a class go beyond exercise. We've found friends.

When you work out with folks three days a week, you encourage one another. You watch out for one another. Being together in a class creates a foxhole effect. The attitude is, "I'm friends with anybody going through this with me."

Our class is fun. We laugh often. We've even set a monthly date to have lunch together.

Not all classes have this result. We've been to classes where folks don't know one another, ignore the instructor, and gossip instead of work out. It does not seem that they share exercise as a common interest.

On the other hand, we've found that the "culture" of a class does not always stay put. People and instructors change or leave. Consequently, we're not keen on just writing something off the list permanently. We might circle back later and try again.

Another benefit of taking a class is structure. The class meets at a set time on scheduled days. We know friends are waiting for us, counting on us to be there to groan and laugh with them. That motivation is very positive.

Finally, we're frugal enough that it seems harder to blow off a class we've paid for. We don't want to "waste" our fee. So, if you're hunting for ways to get up and going, consider taking a class.

Have fun.

Just because we try to be serious about exercising well and regularly does not mean we have to give up having a good time. You can reach out for good times that involve physical activity.

For example, you might consider a trip. Our friend Emma (age 67) is an absolute whiz at swimming. She recently won two firsts, two seconds, two thirds, and a fifth-place ribbon at the National YMCA Competitive Swimming and Diving event in Ft. Lauderdale, Florida.

Yes, I know, she swam with 65-year-old folks. Big deal. Right?

Wrong! I challenge you to swim a hundred-yard individual medley (25 yards each of free form, backstroke, breaststroke, and butterfly) in 1 minute and 29 seconds! The 18- to 24-year-olds took just a tad over 1 minute and 3 seconds to do it.

The point is that Emma challenges herself with achievement goals against swimmers ranked at the national level. Over the past three years, she has entered state events in Michigan (her summer home) and Florida (her winter home) and national events of the Senior Olympics in addition to the YMCA event. In several of these competitions, she set records for the venue and her age group.

Although she competes against others, her biggest challenge has always been to compete against herself. I don't think we've heard a report over the past three years where she has not had the achievement of beating her prior personal-best results. That doesn't happen for every race and every event. But that is her primary goal.

Emma has fun; she gets out and goes to interesting places. She meets interesting people along the way.[12] She travels to challenge herself. And we get to see her newest medals every time she comes to town!

You don't have to look far for competitions to join in a variety of activities:

- The Multiple Sclerosis society in the Mid-South promotes an annual FedEx "Rock-N-Roll" **bike ride** from Memphis to Tunica and back.
- The "Music City Marathon" catches more than 35,000 participants with their **running** shoes on every spring here in Nashville.
- Want to see some great scenery in the Keys? Cart your **kayak** to the "Florida Keys Challenge."
- Throw your **Rollerblades** over your shoulder and head for the "Skate of the Union" in Virginia in June.

But competition is not the only venue that can challenge you to prepare for a "fitness adventure." You might even try an activity you don't normally do.

- Go to a dude ranch and ride a horse.
- Try real farming.
- Canoe trip?
- Ever hiked the Appalachian Trail?
- Go on a Road Scholar adventure.[13]
- Take your grandkids canoeing (hiking, white-water rafting, and so on).

---

12 At the 2013 Senior Olympics, Emma brought home gold and silver. She found inspiration in her impromptu roommate at the event, Laura Roach, who also was a medalist in swimming. Laura is 93!

13 Road Scholar provides what they call "educational adventures." Created by Elderhostel, Inc., these adventures can take you, you and your spouse, or you and your grandchildren on travels filled with learning to the four corners of the world. Check out roadscholar.org.

You might not have to change venues to do different activities. For example, we love taking our grandson on "adventures"—creek-walking, trying disc golf, and checking for frogs at a local nature-center pond. Adding a change of scene transforms an adventure into a "vacation."

Not all these extra activities have to be aerobic or strength-training events. Scheduling one of these extra physical activities can help show you and your family how well you are doing. You should be rewarded for hard work; why not celebrate by showing off the results!

Another reason to mix in a fun event occasionally is to keep things interesting. The treadmill is a lonely place. And, believe it or not, it can get boring. Sputter. Sputter. Cough. Cough. Really?

Find a partner.

Partnerships are important to your success. A partner goes beyond spotting for you or being encouraging. A partnership moves into the area of assessment and challenges, accountability and mutual concern. Partners care about each other's needs, think of ways to be supportive and nurturing, and provide much-needed evaluations a buddy might gloss over.

Make your doctor your partner.

Doctor visits are usually infrequent, likely expensive, and often short. You want to use them effectively. So, be sure to keep your doctor informed about your exercise.

Also, get your physical or wellness exam annually. Early discovery of disease is no guarantee of a cure. But, like exercising six days a week for the rest of your life, being vigilant is one thing you have some control over.

That means you have to step up to the plate. Take responsibility for the thoroughness of each visit. Cover the things that matter to help your doctor have a fuller picture of your health. Prepare for your visits. Have questions you want to ask or a list of things you'd like to learn about. Dr. Daniel G. Amen, in his book *Use Your Brain to Change Your Age*, recommends this list:

- Body Mass Index (BMI)
- Waist-to-height ratio
- Calories needed/calories spent
- Number of fruits and vegetables eaten each day
- Average of hours slept each night
- Blood pressure
- Complete blood count
- General metabolic panel
- HgA1C test for diabetes
- Vitamin D level
- Thyroid levels
- C-reactive protein
- Homocysteine
- Ferritin
- Testosterone
- Lipid panel
- Folic acid and B12 levels
- Syphilis and HIV screenings
- Apolipoprotein E genotype test[14]

I can't go to the drugstore and get a machine that measures my C-reactive protein level. On the other hand, your doctor

14 *Use Your Brain to Change Your Age,* by Daniel G. Amen, Copyright © 2012. Published by Harmony.

can perform specialized tests. You need him or her as a partner if for no other reason than to get the tests done that determine baselines and spot abnormalities.

So, doctor, how's my ferritin level? (Do you know what that is? Do you remember the old commercials for iron deficiency anemia? Bingo! That's it.) I would not have known if I hadn't asked the doctor. So, the first conversation I had with my doctor was, "Is Dr. Amen right? Should we watch these indicators?" The second series of questions I asked was, "What's that for?"

My doctor showed me the tests he did and pointed out how he can tell when there is a problem. As a result, I feel better about having covered all the bases.

Track stuff you can do something about by eating or living right. Some things you can fix, and some you cannot.

This list shows the numbers of deaths annually in the United States attributed to these causes, all of which are completely or largely under your control. Do you have any of these risk factors?

- Smoking: 467,000
- High blood pressure: 395,000
- Overweight-obesity: 216,000
- Inadequate physical activity and inactivity: 191,000
- High blood sugar: 190,000
- High LDL cholesterol: 113,000
- High dietary salt: 102,000
- Low dietary omega-3 fatty acids (seafood): 84,000
- High dietary trans fatty acids: 82,000
- Alcohol use: 64,000 (Alcohol use averted a balance of 26,000 deaths from heart disease, stroke, and diabetes, because moderate drinking reduces risk of these

diseases. But 90,000 alcohol-related deaths from traffic and other injuries, violence, cancers, and a range of other diseases outweigh the benefits.)

- Low intake of fruits and vegetables: 58,000
- Low dietary polyunsaturated fatty acids: 15,000[15]

You don't have to be a statistic. You can do something about the items on this list. You are in charge!

Another reason you want to make your doctor a partner is so you can head the bad guys off at the pass. Early diagnosis is *the* medical miracle cure. A cancer is usually more treatable if discovered early. Early discovery of diabetes might lead to remedies that will keep that nasty disease in check.

One of the possible benefits of improved health is the reduction of medication. The doctor is loath to change something that works. Therefore, he or she is less likely to recommend a medication change spontaneously.

If you keep records, you can watch trends. If you watch trends, you can ask the doctor whether you are ready for medication changes. Showing your trend line of continued improvement might spur the doctor to consider a change.

Record test results

Record results and make lists. Lists show trends. I can see my cholesterol results for the past five years. Because of that, I can tell if I'm winning or losing.

It is true that every one of my cholesterol tests is included in that nice folder the doctor has. I bet, however, that my doctor doesn't shuffle through the pile to learn whether the current reading is an improvement over the last three or four readings.

The same is true of other indicators such as weight, body measurements, and BMI. By keeping records and reviewing them periodically, you can partner with your physician to take action when needed.

---

15 "Smoking, High Blood Pressure and Being Overweight Top Three Preventable Causes of Death in the U.S.," April 27, 2009, press release from the Harvard School of Public Health.

To be sure, if you ask for a reduction because your stats are getting better, your doctor will check his or her records, and not rely on yours. But, if confirmed, changes might be possible. Without keeping track, you might not know to ask, and the doctor might not know to review records.

Another reason for talking things over with your doctor is to report new symptoms. I like to use the "Personal Health Inventory Questionnaire," by Dr. David B. Agus.[16] Dr. Agus recommends completing the form each time you visit your doctor.

Questionnaire results can be extremely revealing and helpful to the doctor. Although all the questions are important, from the standpoint of our concern about exercise and vitality, I found it indicative that six of the first six questions directly relate to items mentioned in this book:

- Overall feeling
- Energy levels
- Schedule (eating and sleeping)
- Breathing
- Exercise tolerance
- Walking

The form includes many other items. All questions relate to energy levels or vitality one way or another. The idea is not to do six and quit; the goal is to point out that the things we talk about in this book are important to a doctor's assessment of your current medical condition.

One final word about this partnership—it is sad but true that disease has randomness. People in good shape die of heart attacks. And people who've never gone out of their way to exercise live full and vibrant lives. Randomness means Russian roulette. Do you want to bet on whether a bullet will

---

16 You will find a link to the questionnaire on his website, davidagus.com. The questionnaire is also repeated in his book, *The End of Illness*, © 2011 by Dr. David B. Agus, published by Free Press, a division of Simon and Shuster, Inc.

come up next time? Neither do I. So, I get a physical every year. You can't be a partner unless you hold up your end.

Your spouse can be a partner.

You may have noticed that much of what I say I do about exercise is also done in partnership with my wife, Crys. She is my buddy, my lifetime companion, and my best friend. We like doing things together.

But we figure we don't have to do everything together. I send her out to ride her horses; she sends me out to do tai chi. I've long since given up riding,[17] and she isn't keen on the slow, dance-like movements of tai chi. But our agreement to exercise means we keep each other accountable, even if we head in opposite directions.

Some mornings, Crys moans about having to go to exercise. I kick her out of bed. Some mornings, I groan about how cold it is and think how wonderful it would be to stay in the nice warm bed. At that point, my wife affixes her permanently frozen feet to the small of my back and reminds me that it can be cold inside as well.

We generally feel better once we're up and going and doing the exercise. I understand the "feel good" portion of the result is likely due to an influx of positive hormones brought on by exercise. We're grateful that only on rare occasions do we moan and groan on the same day. We have found support in the effort that is good for keeping us going.

And, don't even think about starting a nutrition program without involving your partner! Imagine the commentary of the uninitiated: "You're actually gonna eat that stuff!"

My wife and I take turns fixing meals, and we often cook together. She hates grocery shopping as a rule (unless she's

17 Remind me to share with you the "Epic Tale of My Last Ride" sometime.

Together Time

My friend Harry says there are three kinds of marriages:

- *The early marriage—having a large physical component*
- *The middle marriage—rearing the kids*
- *The later marriage—for companionship*

The three kinds can be with different spouses, or all three can be with the same person.

For some couples, the idea of the spouse being underfoot all the time has undermined what could be a very positive third type of marriage. You may have heard the saying, "For better or for worse, but not for lunch!"[18]

From my perspective, the companionship marriage is worth fighting for. It may be hard. I can't say that Crys and I are done struggling with issues, but we've not given up, either. I can't even say that the issues we face are the same as yours.

In our history together, my wife and I have learned one important thing that keeps us going; We've done difficult things before; we can do them again. Getting older is not for the faint-hearted. Having a companion along the way can help.

using the grocery shelves as idea starters for what to fix). I don't mind grocery shopping; I like getting in, getting what's on the list, and getting out. It gets me out of the chair!

It only takes one person to cook, shop, or clean up. On the other hand, by doing these things together, the time is transformed into time together, and we also reinforce our commitment to eating better.

Measure results.

There are many ways to measure results. They all assume that you know why you're measuring and what you want to achieve. Let's talk about goals in general and then about different measuring methods.

Different goal types

The late Zig Ziglar,[19] the motivational speaker, had a famous quotation: "If you aim at nothing, you will hit it every time."

18 *A Couple's Guide to Happy Retirement: For Better or For Worse... But Not For Lunch,* by Sara Yogev, Ph.D. Published by Familius, Second Edition, 2012

19 Author of *Born to Win, Secrets of Closing the Sale,* and others.

At the beginning of our work together, we agreed that doing something—anything—was better than doing nothing. Getting started was the important task. Did you meet that goal? Were you too busy reading this book? Now that we've come away with options, ideas, and plans, we can take the next step and talk about what we want to accomplish.

As I mentioned in Chapter 1, my original goal was to erase that image I have on the mousepad. I didn't want to hang out with that guy anymore. I'm not done with that goal yet. I began where you can begin—imagine yourself the way you want to be. Who is that person? What does she look like? How does he act?

I also know that I'm progressing toward the goal I call "creating a better zoo picture." It is a long-range goal. Keep in mind that "long-range" is different from "impossible," "impractical," or "pie in the sky." On the contrary, I see people who look better than I do in that picture. Though I'm encouraged that my picture is looking better, I can clearly see that others are "getting it right." So, I can too.

A goal also implies what to measure. I'll cross the finish line for this goal when my belt fits properly and not below my belly, my cheeks aren't puffy, and my face doesn't redden with exertion just walking up the stairs.

Crys has a different long-range goal. Some years ago, just after she retired, we went to Barbados and loved it. We wanted to share the adventure with our daughter, son-in-law, and grandson. But at four, our grandson was too young to enjoy many things Crys loves to do, such as swimming in the ocean.

Crys realized that if we wait until our grandson is nine or ten and a strong enough swimmer to enjoy it, she will be nearly seventy when we return to Barbados. So, she set a goal to keep swimming to build her endurance and strength—to be *able* to enjoy that adventure with our family.

Crys' concern for her strength in the water is partly for safety. She is clearly the strongest swimmer in the family, but to stay that way she will have to put in some effort. Her endurance in the water will also contribute to her enjoyment; it will be demanding to keep up with a ten-year-old. She wants a treasured memory with our family.

Unfortunately, just setting the goal does not get results. You have to determine what actions will get you from where you are to where you want to be. I try to evaluate all the steps I've taken on the way to the goal to determine whether I'm headed in the right direction. I'm glad to report positive results:

- Bicycling: Helped with weight loss
- Better nutrition: Helped my weight and my health
- Water aerobics: Helped with endurance and fitness

Crys also has positive results from her lap class. She is moving steadily toward that Barbados trip. Only a year or two left to get ready—go for it, Crys!

Sometimes it is important to set more immediate goals. For example, the first summer my wife and I had our bikes, we decided to bike all the greenways in town sometime during the summer. Sadly, that goal had mixed results. Our first trip was a bust, as we found some greenways did not allow biking.

On the other hand, that goal got us out the door. We went on after-dinner rides in the neighborhood to get ready for longer ones on Saturday. We were active on the bikes, which did us a world of good. Instead of long-range, we'll call this greenway adventure a medium-length goal.

My next medium-length goals are to lose five more pounds and another inch around the belly. I'd like to achieve those before our June vacation.

Our friend Lanette recently gave me another example of a medium-range goal. She was unwilling to go snorkeling on a visit to Costa Rica because it had been too long since she had felt fit enough to try it. She decided that avoiding an activity because of fitness level just would not do. So, she determined that next year she would go snorkeling. To get there, she's started taking swimming lessons with the goal of increasing her endurance and confidence.

It's a good plan. She's not just jumping in with her eyes closed. She's starting with someone who can help her assess and prepare. She also had the second stage sketched out—swimming laps regularly—so she can build to the goal for next year's trip.

The last type of goal is just plain SMART, which is an acronym for

- Specific
- Measurable
- Attainable
- Relevant
- Time-bound

Here are several SMART goals that we might use to help increase our activity level or make our meals healthier:

- In the next seven days, we will prepare dinner at home at least five times.
  Specific: Dinner and home specify time of day and place.
  Measurable: I can count five meals.
  Attainable: Achieving the number is not always easy, but it's possible.
  Relevant: Fewer calories and home cooking are general dietary improvements.

Time-bound: You can measure your success at the end of the period; in this case, the period is a week. I might repeat the same goal, week after week. But by setting the goal each week, I have measurable results that don't float into that hazy place called the future.

- We will do a bicycle ride on a greenway this week.
  Specific: Greenway specifies a venue. Adding a location name might be beneficial.
  Measurable: Only one thing to do—ride.
  Attainable: Only impossible if it rains every day.
  Relevant: Biking is a good activity for me.
  Time-bound: We have just a week; better get out there while the sun is out.

If you need some SMART ideas to get started, look at Appendix A. There you will find more examples, plus details about what constitutes a SMART goal.

Progress can be measured. You won't know whether you make much headway or lose ground unless you measure where you stand. In general, there are four things to consider:

1. The big picture
2. The little things
3. You and your heart rate
4. Personal activity monitors

The big picture

I gained a year yesterday; it was my birthday. But today, according to the RealAge Test,[20] I'm 3.8 years younger!

---

20 Realage.com, Dr. Oz's website. Check out the RealAge Test. Sign up through sharecare.com for their weekly newsletters too. The topics are helpful, but perhaps the biggest help is the regular reminder that you can do things to better ensure your health.

You need to check out this free online assessment tool. After entering answers to a survey of your current health, feelings, diet, and fitness, you are rewarded with an estimate of your biological age compared with your chronological age.

It worked! Yesterday, I was a year older according to the calendar. Today, I'm almost four years younger! I plan to take the RealAge test on my birthday every year. It will give me an overview estimate of how well I'm doing. It provides a big-picture approach, the bird's-eye view.

I'm also going to do the Vitality Compass survey from the Blue Zones people. A Blue Zone is an area in the world where people live vibrant and active lives into their 90s and 100s. Besides promoting the things these longevity stars share, the website[21] lets you take their Vitality Compass.

After entering answers to questions about health background, outlook, flexibility, eating habits, social community, lifestyle, and environment, the survey gave me a biological age of 59. Whoopee! I *like* this survey. It's going on the yearly list too. You can't beat gaining eight years.

A yearly physical is also an important overview tool. Among other things, this annual visit gives your doctor an excuse to measure all those indicators listed earlier in the section on partnering. The annual checkup is a free service offered to Medicare[22] recipients. If you are on Medicare, many tests are also free to you because of their preventive nature.

---

21 BlueZones.com. Check out the Vitality Compass. A word to the wise: Take the test just before you have dessert. I had cherry pie for my birthday and leftovers several days more. Unfortunately, the survey asked how many servings of sugars I'd had during the past week. Oops! I limit dessert to once a week or less the rest of the time. I'll be smarter about the sugar thing next year.

22 Some Medicare advantage plans take extra steps to encourage prevention, including having an annual checkup. Use the website or booklets they provide to help your planning.

The little things

Similarly, you need to develop a long-range list with your doctor for other tests:

- Mammograms
- Bone mass measurements
- Colonoscopy

Of course, there are more. Work with your doctor, and ask what tests you should have and when. All items on the lists above need to be discussed and, if needed, scheduled.

With all this testing going on, are you beginning to see how some of your retirement time will be spent? Many of these measurements are infrequent. And, sometimes, a single measure means more to the doctor if given in context. A single blood pressure reading might look high, for example. But given how blood pressure can fluctuate during the day, it might make more sense to the doctor if he or she knew where this measurement fit in a graph of measurements made at different times during the day.

Give yourself a measurement triad. For three days, track your blood pressure every two hours and create a chart of the result. The chart should compare the three days by hour of the day. The next time you go to the doctor and your blood pressure is checked, give the doctor the graph for comparison. Unless you want to go down to the pharmacy every two hours to use their machine, you might want to purchase a blood pressure cuff.

This plan seems like a lot of trouble for one measurement, until you consider the consequences. High blood pressure is the second-leading cause of death in the U.S.

You can also create graphs equally helpful for

- Sugar levels (particularly if you are diabetic)
- Weight
- Heart rate

And more. Again, talk with your doctor. What would help?

You and your heart rate

Another reason to do detailed and frequent measurement is to determine stress levels during activity. Chris Crowley is a dictator about monitoring your heart rate during exercise.[23] The point is obvious—you can't know how well you are doing until you pay attention. With strenuous exercise, paying attention to heart rate is critical.

Paying attention means that you know what should be done, what *your* body can do, and what is happening during exercise. Decades of measurements for thousands of athletes provide a profile to follow. Because of extensive research, *Younger Next Year* author Chris Crowley can detail what effort levels to achieve if you want to increase your stamina and fitness—what he calls building your aerobic base. The only way to know whether you are winning or losing is to measure. The measurement that works is heart rate.

Heart rate is only an effective measure if you know what yours should be. The measure is called the target heart rate. You can use different calculations to find the specific number that fits you and to set different workout levels.[24]

---

23 *Younger Next Year, Live Strong, Fit, and Sexy—Until You're 80 and Beyond*, by Chris Crowley and Henry S. Lodge, M.D. Copyright ″ 2007 by Chris Crowley and Henry S. Lodge. Published by Workman Publishing Company.

24 Usually calculated as 220 minus your age, 85% (or more) of calculated result is your anaerobic level. When exercising, I call this full tilt; it should be done only after warming up (and then, only after your doctor gives the OK). High endurance is 70%–85% of target. At the long and slow rate (50%–70%), you should be able to sustain activity for hours if you are aerobically fit. You only want to try full tilt when you can measure results, and you know how to work safely up to it. Full tilt is *not* for Day 1. Going 100% of target rate is *not* advisable.

I find the numbers are good for me. One of the classes I take is a particularly active water aerobics class. The instructor takes us into that anaerobic level gradually and has us measure heart rate at the end of the anaerobic activity. I have to work hard to get into the 90% range set for me by the calculation method. (See footnote.)

My friend Dave, however, says those numbers derived from the calculation are much too low for him. His heart rate easily goes above levels I find a strain. Dave has not had bypass surgery, and he is in better shape than I am.

The moral here: Know thyself.

The only way to get personally accurate numbers and, therefore, be able to set appropriate goals, is to ask your doctor for a stress test. Again, with your doctor as your partner, you can talk about the test, the need, and your course of action. Figure out a plan that works for you.

You might want to consider using a heart-rate monitor while exercising. At $100, this device could pay off in big ways. On your own, you can't tell when your heart rate spikes, for example. You want to stop what you're doing when that happens. I understand that unless the spiking begins to happen regularly, it is somewhat normal, but without the device you can't monitor what's going on inside your heart.

When you start your program, you definitely want to stay way below your 90% (anaerobic) level. When you've achieved a higher endurance level, you can push that limit. Even then, you want to know when you've gotten there. A monitor can tell you when you approach these performance thresholds.

A monitor can also help you know your resting heart rate and your recovery heart rate. Both these measures are significant indicators of health and fitness.

Take your doctor's advice about the monitor and the readings. Your doctor might be able to recommend the correct device for you. Before using it, be sure you know target heart-rate ranges for different levels of activity.

Personal activity monitors

If you are interested in monitoring general activity, cool tools are available for that as well. The measurement tool I use is called Fitbit,[25] a little fob I carry in my pocket or strap to my wrist at bedtime. It tracks a variety of things:

- Steps taken today
- Number of floors climbed today
- Miles traveled today
- Calories burned today (based on BMI)

This data is collected automatically through the wireless connection in my home. Through an application on my computer, the data is sent to a database in a web application. After tracking all this, the webpage shows me a general report on my day's activity level.

Activity

updated 14 mins ago

6736 steps taken today   **67%** of goal of **10,000**

6 floors climbed today   **60%** of goal of **10**
You have climbed: The Tallest Dinosaur ★

3.1 miles traveled today   **62%** of goal of **5.00**

1284 calories burned   **59%** of goal of **2,184**

522 active score ⓘ   **52%** of goal of **1,000**

---

25 fitbit.com

Not bad for 11 A.M. I have a good start for the day and time remaining to make the goals.

Goals make using this device beneficial to me. I can personalize the goals shown (such as 10,000 steps taken today). When I got the device, I wanted to establish a baseline. How active am I? How sedentary? So, for now, I'm seeing how well I do against the defaults the Fitbit folks provided.[26] When I'm done taking stock, I'll start setting goals that I can live with by establishing methods to go with the goals. Here is the plan:

- To be less sedentary, I plan to get out of my desk chair at intervals and walk a prescribed route. SMART goals will come in handy.
- I haven't figured out about the floors climbed yet. There is a slight hill in front of my house. Fitbit translates hills into floors climbed. I'll take periodic breaks and walk up and down the hill.

Fitbit tracks more items than I have discussed. The "active score" is a calculation that gives the user a summary. Do nothing and get an active score of 0. Be active and your score climbs into the three-digit range. I haven't found out yet how much you have to do to get into the four-digit range.

The program tracks different levels of activity: Sedentary, Lightly Active, Fairly Active, and Very Active. A chart by percent of each of these levels gives you another overview of how well you are doing. The program lets you record foods eaten and add your activities. (Because the device won't go in water, I have to add the water aerobics class.) It tracks calories in and calories expended. It also monitors sleep patterns and other health indicators.

---

26 It has been six months since I wrote this. When I compare my weekly stats from the past month to the first month, I've found my average went up by 10,000 steps a week. Apparently just watching what I do every day makes a difference.

The number of similar devices is growing:

- **Striiv**
- **NewYu**
- **FIT CORE** Armband[27]
- **Direct Life** from Phillips
- **BodyMedia Fit**
- **Gruve** by Muve
- Motorola **KORE**
- **myTrek** by Scosche
- **Replay** by Switch2Health
- **Basis** by Basis Science, Inc.
- **muCoach** by Adidas
- **Up** by Jawbone

Here are some important factors to consider when you review devices:

- What does it record?

  If you're trying to get better at cycling, a computer for your bicycle might be a good choice. If you need coaching, you might prefer the devices that provide personalized planning. What are your goals?
- How is the data reported?

  On the device?

  On a computer (through the web or an application)?

  On a cell phone or tablet computer?

  These options are often mutually exclusive. You can only see the data on a phone, tablet computer, or the device itself.

27 Su Reid St. John, senior fitness editor at health.com, reviews the first three listed along with Fitbit on their fitness blog.

- Can I really transport it?

    A keychain device might show a male audience bias, as men are more likely to carry key chains in pockets. Some devices look like watches or armbands. One is worn as a necklace. (Would that be a female audience bias?)

- Is there a social component?

    Some allow you to build a community of encouragement. Some charge a fee and offer networking features. My buddy Mike, who lives two states away, and I track how many steps we've taken; our daily Fitbit report shows both of us the last seven days' worth.

- Does it come with coaching?

    Some charge a yearly fee for helping develop personal fitness plans and, oh, by the way, a device comes with it. Others start with the device, and you can get add-on support of various kinds.

- What are the special features?

    The BodyMedia Fit vibrates to warn you when you've been sitting too long at a stretch, for example.

- How is data uploaded (if necessary)?

    USB, wireless, Bluetooth, or audio jack (for smartphone connections) are also usually mutually exclusive.

The goal of all these personal devices is to help track occasional activity and summarize it in a way that portrays a bigger picture. Because you need to get out of your chair and move around, you'll want to invent ways to be more active, like taking the stairs instead of the elevator or parking farther away from the store so you can walk.

Even though you might be doing a bang-up job of getting in a strenuous workout every day, the advantage can be whittled away by sitting the rest of the time. Thorn Klosowski says more than six hours of sitting a day can increase your risk of heart disease, shorten your life, and increase your chances of some types of cancer. "Even people who exercise regularly are subject to the negative health effects of prolonged periods of sitting."[28]

Try some ways to add exercise to your daily routine:

- At work you can
  - o Park near the back of the parking lot so you can walk farther.
  - o Stand to visit the filing cabinet instead of rolling your chair.
  - o Walk over and talk to a coworker instead of sending him or her an email.
  - o Take the scenic route to the kitchen or bathroom.
  - o Walk at lunch or break time.

- At your desk, you can get out of that chair and move for short periods. Here's a good one-minute workout[29]:
  - o Stand.
  - o March in place for twenty seconds.
  - o Reach down and touch your toes repeatedly for twenty seconds.
  - o Wander around and pick up or reorganize items for the last twenty seconds.

You might wish to explore two other categories of devices: ones that are exercise-specific and smartphone apps.

I mentioned my friend Dave earlier. Bicycling is his aerobic exercise of choice. He got an Edge device made by Garmin. It attaches to his bike and measures speed, distance, time, calories

---

28 "How Sitting All Day Is Damaging Your Body and How You Can Counteract It," by Thorin Klosowski, lifehacker.com, January 16, 2012.

29 "How Sitting All Day Is Damaging Your Body and How You Can Counteract It," by Thorin Klosowski, lifehacker.com, January 16, 2012.

burned, altitude, climb, and descent, and records data for review. He particularly likes that the device records cadence.

With Garmin's "Courses" feature, Dave can compare performance between tries at the same route. And, with a compatible meter, the device will record a history of heart rate during exercise. If you are a cyclist, you will want to review the scores of measuring devices available.

The number of apps for smartphones grows almost daily. I have an "iPhone-centric" knowledge of applications for these devices, so I know that iPhone offers a whole set of apps. For example, I use the Strava app to track my bicycle rides. Distance and time are exactly what I'm interested in and that's all I use it for. Pedometers, body fat calculators, a fitness builder, and weight improvement apps are also available.

You owe it to yourself to check out what's available as a stand-alone device or on your phone. The American Heart Association reports this encouraging news:

> *Overweight and obese adults who used an electronic diary program on a personal digital assistant did better at staying on diet and physical activity programs....*
>
> *People using the device, which provided tailored dietary and exercise feedback messages, were more successful in adhering to five treatment factors for weight loss:*
>
> - *attending group sessions;*
> - *meeting daily calorie goals;*
> - *meeting daily fat intake goals;*
> - *reaching weekly exercise goals; and*
> - *monitoring eating and exercise.*
>
> *Those using the electronic devices did significantly better than those using a paper diary....*[30]

30 "Overweight, Obese Adults Use Electronic Device to Stick to Diet, Exercise," American Heart Association's Epidemiology and Prevention/Nutrition, Physical Activity and Metabolism 2012 Scientific Sessions, March 15, 2012.

Track results.

Measuring is only the beginning. Tracking is also important for several reasons. With a good tracking system you can:

- Catch trends.
- Detect anomalies.
- Note due dates.
- Transport data.

Catch trends.

I have a little database that I use to record

- Immunizations
- Procedures (carpal tunnel surgery, bypass, and so on)
- Drugs and supplements
- Weight
- Height
- Body measurements (chest, belly, waist, and hips)
- Test results (cholesterol, blood pressure, BMI)

Many of these results are general indicators of well-being. Most, however, are directly driven by how I exercise and eat.

I review the data before a doctor visit. Most doctors will require a current list of medications. So, I check the list to be sure it is accurate, print a copy for my wallet, and print a copy for the visit. My medication list also includes the one item I'm allergic to. Thus, I have a way to get that noted on my chart.

As I prepare to go to the doctor, I mark any prescriptions due a refill. I also note any brand names so I can ask about the availability of generics. I check for any prescriptions that might be candidates for an over-the-counter substitution.

A doctor friend recommended that I remind you to take your medications, bottles and all, to your internist (general practitioner, primary care physician) annually. You might also want to take the little pill cases along, too. Why? So the doctor can see that you

- Take morning pills in the morning and nighttime pills at night
- Actually received the drug recommended
- Take the correct dose
- Use drugs prescribed by another doctor

All kinds of *bad things can happen* if any of these are incorrect and your doctor doesn't know about them.

Your doctor can also check for possible interactions. If you're like me, not all your meds come from the same pharmacy. So, these interactions won't be checked anywhere else but the doctor's office.

In checking prescriptions, I also check trends. For example, I'll look at the cholesterol record over the last two years to learn whether I'm winning or losing. If I'm winning, and the levels are well within goals, I'll consider asking the doctor for a reduction, substitution, or drug elimination.

If I'm losing, I make sure to call this concern to the doctor's attention. The doctor can glance at my list and spot something that might need to change. Hunting through stacks of paper in his folder might not net the same result.

To be sure, my doctor will check his records to see that my numbers are correct. But having my list eliminates effort and saves time, which I want spent during the visit discussing options.

Detect anomalies.

My lists help spot anomalies—the list can suggest something that shouldn't be there. Sudden weight gain? Loss? Sugar level or PSA level spikes?

Note due dates.

Finally, I check due dates. When was the last colonoscopy? Flu shot? Pneumonia vaccination? I will be sure to call these things to the doctor's attention.

In Appendix B, I've created a starter list of the information you can record. Your list will likely vary if you have health issues different from or in addition to mine, so add and subtract as needed.

Before I retired, I was a database developer (Translation: A geek who played with computers). So, I use a database to keep my list. If you want to go low-tech, get a yellow legal pad and a ruler. Write the headings across the top of the page and use the ruler to mark column divisions. *Voilà!* A medium-tech solution would be to use a spreadsheet on your computer.

Let's talk specifics a little. Here is part of my measurement list. As I mentioned earlier, I'm interested in my waist size so that's what I'm showing:

Date	Waist
Mar 20, 2010	42
Sep 4, 2010	40
Sep 7, 2011	41
Mar 1, 2012	39

You can see immediately the advantage of having a list. I obviously had some ups and downs. But keeping track has helped me achieve the range I sought.

Originally we were told that a waist measurement of 40 inches or more for men was a bad thing. The apple-shaped man was in for trouble. So, I've worked very hard to get below the 40 inches. Sadly, while I pedaled my bike and ran around doing water aerobics, the rules changed. It turns out that a

40-inch measurement was less a problem for a man taller than I am.

So, now, the rule suggests that your waist should be less than half your height in inches. A ratio of waist to height is fair to all no matter how tall you are. Because I'm shorter than 78 inches (twice 39), I still have a problem. I was very proud of myself when I finally made the old goal, but now, I'll make a new one.

Transport data.

Collecting and maintaining records about your well-being has become so prevalent and pervasive, it is referred to by its initials:

PHR (Personal Health Record)

A variety of programs will help you collect such data. Evaluation of options goes way beyond the scope of this document. I've included a summary in Appendix B.

Much of the data currently collected in PHR systems is static. The fact that your mother had breast cancer is not likely to change. Besides your family medical history, your basic information—your address and other contact information, even your list of medications—is unlikely to change often.

So, basically, your work to use this type of record keeping is front-loaded. It takes you a while to get it recorded, but it does not take too long to keep up with the changes.

The big advantage to having all that data in one place is the ability to get it to another place. I'm sorry to say that, though these PHR systems will let you export the data, very few doctors can currently load that data into their computer, except by typing it again, which means filling out the doctor's form. It is much easier to fill out those forms at the doctor's office if you have a list to refer to, and you can print the list from PHR systems.

For You

To get help with taking exercise seriously, check out the website:

www.retireto.info/be-able/bookresources/

I've included the SMART goals from Appendix A plus an additional fifteen in different categories. These are formatted so you can edit out the ones you don't want, highlight ones you want, add your own, and print them.

I've also included a chart you can post. It highlights the rule: Exercise one hour a day, six days a week for the rest of your life. It also shows the six days and gives you room to record your schedule. Post it as well. Every bit of motivation helps.

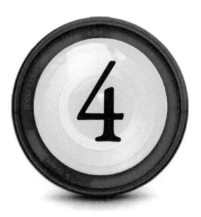

Get Good Food

There are great excuses for not eating better. I know because I've used many of them. See if you recognize any:

- Who knows what's good for you? One day you can't eat this, but the next day you can. Coffee is bad for you; coffee is good for you. Stay away from sweets, but chocolate is good for you. Vegetables are great, but some don't count.
- I tried that diet—it didn't work.
- Why would they sell the stuff if it weren't good for you? Isn't that illegal?
- I'm a terrible cook. So, we eat out a lot.
- I travel frequently, so I can't eat well.

What follows is a list of actions I find helpful for eating better. You might have found other things that work for you.

- Take small bites.
- Eat out—carefully.
- Rediscover home.
- Watch what you eat.
- Avoid hunger.
- Tame cravings.
- Know your food.

Take small bites.

Although there are all kinds of things you can do to practice healthier eating, I think Crys and I have discovered the truth of the matter—you can't fix everything at once. So, largely, we've tried one thing at a time until it becomes the new normal. Here are a couple of examples:

I like crackers with my soup. I (still) probably use too many, but I'm now using whole-wheat crackers. Whole wheat, you understand, is better for you than plain white crackers. I've found that I've grown to prefer the whole-wheat variety. So much so that when my wife succumbed to a sale and purchased a box of white crackers recently, I commented on how tasteless they seem now. I've found the same is true of whole-wheat pasta.

So, although it took some time to get into the whole-wheat thing, by tackling it all by itself, we were able to switch from using foods made from white, processed flour. We started with crackers, moved to pasta, and now we are changing our bread choices.

Another example has to do with sugar and sugar substitutes. For me, the problem is old habits that were formed when I was a child. I put sugar on my cereal and on my fruit. Adding sugar was standard, and nobody said a thing. The people who catch me doing that now think I'm very strange.

So, what could I do about it? I started using sugar substitutes. Everybody knows there are no calories in sugar substitutes. And, for a long time, that was my nutritional goal—to avoid calories. Now I know other things are at stake.

Your body does not know how to metabolize sugar substitutes. Therefore, they can't be good for you. And, because you metabolize sugar too rapidly, you still need to avoid it (diabetes, don't you know). Now, I try to eliminate the substitute stuff altogether. What do you substitute for a substitute?[31]

I'm working at it one item at a time. With cereal, I'm trying not to add sugar and use only cereal products in which sugar is not in the top three ingredients. Because of the nutritional concerns against high fructose corn syrup, I try to stay away from anything that includes it in the ingredients list.

We've long since given up colas and other soft drinks. But I do get tired of just plain water and want to treat myself occasionally to a liquid with some taste. I haven't found a good alternative. Although I drink coffee without sugar, I prefer my tea sweet. See the problem? My friend Erin, who is also a personal trainer and exercise specialist, suggested her trick of adding pure cherry or lime juice to water. Hmm, maybe I'll give that a go.

Well, that's it. We're still working at it. One ingredient. One product. One item at a time. Steadily forward wins the race. So, instead of trying to tackle all the issues at once, we've started with small steps. As sci-fi writer Robert Heinlein suggests, divide your "mountain" into a large number of small parts. In nutrition, where do the small parts come from? Food groups.

---

31 A nutritionist recommended *The American Dietetic Association Food and Nutrition Guide* as a good resource for diabetics.

In many American kitchens there are four main food groups:

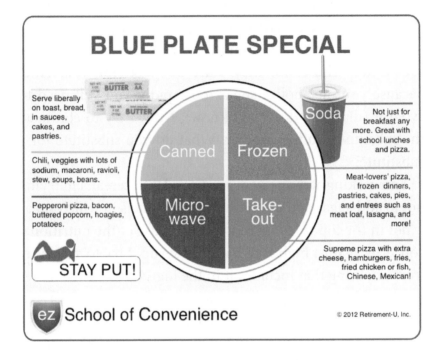

Canned, Frozen, Microwave, Take-Out. Oops! That's the old chart. These days we're trying to do a little better.

Nutritionists have debated a new food-group chart over the past few years. If you've not seen the new one, you might want to look up some details. On the next page is the version from Harvard,[32] which includes descriptions of each item:

---

32 Used by permission of Harvard Health Publications. Excerpted from Harvard Health Blog, September 14, 2011, copyright © 2011, Harvard University. Harvard Health Publications does not endorse any products or medical procedures.

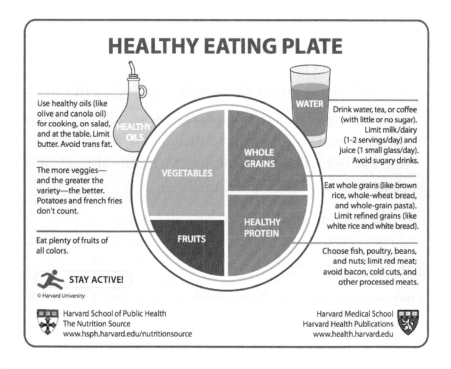

The idea here is to pick a category and start. You can develop all kinds of healthful goals from just the items shown here. For example:

- Let's eat fish twice a week.
- Can we cook with olive oil instead?
- I'll fix brown rice next time.

Note that grains on this chart take much less room than they did on the chart we grew up using. Vegetables and fruits occupy half the plate! That is the point: Start your planning around using vegetables and fruit and reduce the intake of meats and grains. Start your meal preparation with ingredients lower on the food chain.

If you examine the ingredients listed on this chart, you will find a wealth of examples just waiting for a SMART goal series.

- I will eat a banana for breakfast tomorrow and some cantaloupe for dinner.
- This week I'm buying brown rice instead of white.
- I will ask my grocer about good fish choices this week.

A SMART goal overview appears in Appendix A; I've also included several sample goals related to food selection.

But the bottom line, according to healthful-food guru Michael Pollan, is really quite simple:

Eat food. Mostly plants. Not too much.[33]

Eat out—carefully.

After our daughter left home, and my wife and I were fully invested in very active, demanding careers, it was much easier to cope with the pressures by eating out. You know how the discussion went:

- What if we stop and pick up something?
- Do you really want to cook?
- Do we have anything in the fridge?

You can make wise choices eating out. But you need to practice making these choices, or you can succumb again to large portions, high cholesterol, sugar, salt, and deep-fried offerings. You can make better selections:

- Go for baked or broiled options (skip fried).
- Select small salads or vegetables without sauces over large meat portions.
- Share your meal with a companion or use a takeout box.
- Watch for "heart-healthy" menu options.

---

33 *Food Rules: An Eater's Manual,* by Michael Pollan. Copyright (c) 2009. Published by Penguin Books.

- Plan and use online sources for menu information. Select an optimal list of restaurants ahead of time. When the need arises, use a restaurant on your list.
- Plan with preselected food choices.
- Don't look at the wonderful food pictures on the menu! Instead, pay attention to the new calorie counts that should appear in restaurant menus soon.

There are exceptions to everything. One restaurant's salad might be quite high in calories. However, my bet is—and it is a bet—that the restaurant that serves a salad high in calories serves meat portions even more out of kilter.

Overall, you can probably prepare better meals at home and often do so less expensively. With a little planning, you may even be able to eat sooner at home than you could if you stopped at a restaurant. So, let's explore some ins and outs of cooking at home.

Rediscover home.

A plan from my past:

> When I was a teenager at home for the summer, my mom decided my sister and I needed meal preparation instruction. She told us that because we were home doing nothing while she went to work all day, the least we could do was have dinner ready when she got home. "What's so hard about that?" she would say, and she gave us her cooking plan: "Just pick a meat from the freezer, cook some kind of potato, and open a can of vegetables."

Hmm, I have to give Mom credit, though. The "can" of vegetables was usually one prepared by my grandmother from her garden.

This plan had a couple of good things. The first item of note is that Mom's plan contained only one **processed food**, if you count my grandmother's contribution. Watch processed foods carefully; they often contain "secret" ingredients to add flavor or act as preservatives.[34]

Shop on the outside aisles of your grocery where the fresh and not-processed foods are displayed. Avoid processed foods by making 80% of your choices from the "ring around the grocery." Stores generally stock that way to coax buyers into walking through the aisles to visit the whole store. When you're standing in front of the milk, where are the vegetables? On the far side of the store from where you are, of course!

A second good thing about Mom's plan was that she shopped and **stocked ahead**. I understand that you might be tempted to grab your net bag and stop at the produce place on your way home (not!). We're in a hurry here! We're hungry.

Mom didn't particularly care which protein we used at any time. She just made sure it didn't take any extra effort to get to it. It was in the freezer. You can do the same thing with a plan.

My friend Paul found himself a single parent at a time in his life when he was also a very busy executive. He did not have time to plan meals. So, he made a two-week meal plan once and didn't worry about it again. "We always had beef roast on Sunday. I counted on the leftovers for dinner Tuesday night and beef slices for a lunch or two." This plan minimized complications for shopping and preparation and stopped the ever-present set of choices needed when you find yourself without a plan.

If you have trouble with meal planning, know your grocer. Grocers are often good sources of quick meal-planning tips. Some groceries even have recipe cards and isolate the

---

34 Alas, even Gramma's canned vegetables probably had too much salt and her fruits too much sugar. But they were good!

ingredients for a particular recipe in one place (for your shopping convenience). That does not mean the grocer always has the healthiest choices available, so you have to evaluate. But these days, she is mindful and attentive to healthful alternates, so it doesn't hurt to ask. Is there a leaner meat choice or a different sauce? Do I have to fry it?

By knowing your grocer, you can also begin to learn how items are stocked and when. The produce is freshest when? The fish comes in how? And when he knows you're interested in economy, your grocer can steer you to a less expensive tasty choice. He'll often give you unsolicited information because he knows the news he has (like a sale price) is of interest to you—you've inquired previously.

Alas, I can't help you in the meal-planning department. I am not Paul. Besides, I favor a little more variety. My wife and I are just not good at planning meals to the point that if it is Tuesday, we know we're having fish. The tradeoff means we have daily choices to make.

We try to solve the problem the same way my mom did— stock ahead and limit our choice for a meal to what is in the freezer or cupboard. If we haven't had fish this week, that fact informs our decision. But that only works if it's on hand.

Mom's meal preparation plan also leaves a few things to be desired. You might be able to tell "I'm a meat-and-potatoes man" just from her plan. So, one of the first shortcomings is the high proportion of carbohydrates in the plan. These days we try to **limit carbohydrates**; in particular, we try to limit white potatoes to one meal a week (and my wife keeps trying to sneak in sweet potatoes instead of Irish).

Mom's plan was low on vegetables. Today we often go for raw vegetables. And we try not to go a day without eating at least **three servings of vegetables**. We concentrate on vegetables with bright colors (peppers, broccoli, tomatoes); I understand that the brightly colored ones are generally more nutritious.

What about fruit in Mom's plan? Oops! I forgot. Mom made sure the standard items were stocked. We could have fruit cocktail (from a can) or canned peaches (from Gramma) for dessert once in a while. There you go. Problem solved?

Maybe not! These days we favor raw fruit when available and try to get at least **two servings of fruit a day**. If you notice in the food chart, fruit juice is not a recommended substitute for real fruit. Because fruit juice is processed, it doesn't have the same nutritional value and might contain additives that are not advised. Then, too, the meat of the fruit has fiber and nutrients often discarded to make juice; even the items with pulp don't have the same nutritional value.

Fresh fruits and vegetables might be difficult to get or, in a sense, to swallow. Some people just don't like or eat raw vegetables. Then, canned is better than none, and sometimes, frozen has more nutrients than fresh.

A consistent pattern Crys and I've developed is to make **more nutritious substitutes**. We use

- Virgin olive oil to make grilled cheese sandwiches. And the cheese these days is likely to be fat free.
- Blue chips or pita chips instead of potato chips.
- Salsa on a baked potato instead of butter or sour cream.

Watch what you eat.

When Crys and I started the twelve-week fitness program at our wellness center, we were introduced to the food journal. Since then, using a log has become a visible part of our lives.

Here is a completed sample of the food journal we created for our use:

Recruit exercise buddies for the variety of activities you do.		1/3
Breakfast (time:) Oats walnuts yogurt banana	Morning Snack	D, calcium **Limit:** Red meat, Butter, Sweets, White Foods, Salt
Lunch (time:) Bean soup Whole wheat crackers butter	Afternoon Snack dark chocolate square	Lowfat Dairy ☑☐ ☑☐ Nuts, Seeds ☑☑ ☑☑ Beans ☑☐
Dinner (time:) spaghetti cheese salad cranberries sauce bread pecans turkey garlic butter dressing	Evening Snack coconut cake	Fish, Poultry, Eggs ☑☐ ☐☐ Healthy Oils/MUFA ☑☐ ☐☐ Fruits ☑☑ ☐☐
Exercise = 15 minutes ☑☑ ☑☑☐☐☐☐ water aerobics retirement-u.com	Water = 8 oz ☑☑☑☑☑☐ ☐☐	Vegetables ☑☑☑ ☐☐☐ Whole Grains ☑☑☑☐☐ ☐☐

As you fill in the details on the left, you can check off items in the right column. You can see walnuts for breakfast and pecans during dinner in the description area; on the right, "Nuts, Seeds" has two check marks.

Do you see the slight spacing after the first two fruit boxes and after the first three vegetable boxes? The number of boxes to the left represents the recommended amounts. So, we show two fruits and three vegetables. We also show a minimum of a half-hour of exercise and one low-fat dairy product. All this, of course, is for one day.

Using a journal like this has several advantages. For one thing, the records are important for doing a self-assessment such as the ones on RealAge or BlueZones. In the past, they've asked questions such as how many nut servings have you had in the past month or dairy servings in the past week. Without some record, you are guessing. I have a terrific memory, but it is very short. I could not answer without having the details stored.

For another thing, you can start setting goals and tracking achievements. It is good to know you should eat three vegetables a day. It is better to know that you did! (If I have to eat vegetables, at least I want credit for it.) The process is called accountability. I also take these journals to my doctor and cardiologist. When they ask about eating habits—and they have—I can show them.

You can get a copy of the latest food journal on the website for this book (www.retireto.com/be-able/bookresources). I say, "latest," because we continue to improve things. For example, it seems important to know how you felt when you ate—sad, happy, nervous, bored? At the end of the day (or the week, month), you'll know more about yourself, and you can make better food choices. We might add that to our journal.

You can find other food journals on the Internet by typing "food journal" in a search page. Other journals can help you track calories, carbs, fat, and so on. Crys and I would prefer not to measure calories all the time. So, I can't help you much about the ins and outs of calorie counting. But other websites can. MyPlate and Calorie King are two good examples.

The point: Pick a food log based on what you want or need to track. If you are diabetic, you will be much more concerned about glycemic index than other folks will. As a diabetic, you'll find it important to identify why your glucose levels rise or fall sometimes. Journaling can help with these things.

Follow these two rules:

Don't lie. You're only cheating yourself if you keep your doctor or your dietitian in the dark. You must record everything you eat. You must be accurate. If you don't reach your goals today, you have tomorrow to try again.

Write as you go. Again, the memory thing. My memory is too short so it makes sense to make notes after the meal. But this rule is also important for snack times. Don't forget the little things.

According to an article by Dr. Oz and Dr. Roizen:

Out of nearly 1,700 overweight people on a six-month weight loss program, those who kept a daily food journal lost twice as much weight as those who didn't keep a journal.[35]

Another way to watch what we eat is to watch what we buy. Crys and I shop together, cook together, and, in general, keep an eye on each other. As my wife says, "You really want that?" or "Do you need three of those?" All terrible questions! It's not called "for better or worse" for nothing.

I'm told that some people can't stand keeping journals or being so structured. Fine. If you can't, don't. But I want you to think of ways to pay attention. Knowing what and how well you're doing is central to being able to do something about a problem. Be watchful. Learn what you do. Take small steps to improve on what you find.

Avoid hunger.

The food journal shown previously has room for three **snacks** a day. The concept behind this approach is simple. If you eat small but more frequent meals, you will be less hungry and therefore won't overeat. A great idea.

But some people can't keep to the plan. Eating too much at snack time is too easy. It's OK to eat too much at snack time as long as you don't eat as much as you would otherwise at the following meal. For some folks (like me), snacks just

---

35 RealAge Tip published August 22, 2010, at RealAge.com

grow. Can't eat just one! In other words, Plan A doesn't work for some folks.

It is a time-honored tradition to go for Plan B when the first plan fails. Plan B starts with the same general idea—eat a snack to keep from getting too hungry by mealtime. The difference in Plan B is that you don't have to do a snack between two meals if the meals are relatively close.

Generally, breakfast and lunch are closer together than lunch and dinner. If the meals are more than four hours apart, consider having a small snack at the fourth hour (or thereabouts).

A second part of the plan is to treat a snack as normal. A snack is not a reward. A snack is not a treat. It is just fuel. Eat, and be done. Do the same snack every time.

- Eight pita chips with hummus
- An apple or orange
- A small bunch of grapes
- A small handful of walnuts

Add a glass of water, and all of these ideas are great snacks. Go for 100 calories or less. Don't go for the 100-calorie bag of cookies or chips from the grocery or vending machine if you can avoid it—remember the processed-food danger.

I've always had a problem with **portion control**. It is too easy to "supersize it," even when cooking at home. Because potatoes are my particular hobgoblin, I try to take particular care with them. When Crys and I prepare for ourselves, we've gone to serving one or two small new potatoes instead of one of the giant economy size. Here are other tips:

- Use smaller plates, and don't pile them high.

- Leave some food on your plate. I'm told that you will eat less if there is evidence around suggesting you already ate a lot.
- Serve the salad first, and don't clear the salad plates.
- Don't serve family style. Build and deliver dinner plates. (I feel more comfortable doing this at meals when we're only serving the two of us.)
- If you must have seconds, take more salad or vegetables.
- Eat slowly. We had twenty-five-minute lunch periods in high school; since then, eating quickly has largely been the norm for me, and when I have more time to eat, I eat more! I'm trying to do better.

Tame cravings.

When my wife gets into the middle of a project, she eats. This compulsion is not from hunger, but from stress. It's akin to chewing your nails or eating popcorn at the movies. Two basic synergies seem to be involved:

- **Learned behavior**: We enjoy foods that make us feel good (sugary, fatty, salty foods stimulate endorphins). So we look for other foods or eat more of the old items to bring back the good feelings.
- **Environment**: If you live in a neighborhood where the only readily available food choices are bad ones, you have little choice. If you live in such a neighborhood, you might also be without the means to get to an alternate location. It's a triple whammy because once you've learned to eat the foods available, that behavior might maintain the upper hand even if the food options improve.

The solutions to these tendencies are avoidance and control. Easier said than done! Consider these options:

- **Don't keep bad food choices around.** If you can't help bingeing on a particular candy, don't buy it anymore. Don't stock potato chips, hot dogs, pastries, and on and on.

- **Don't go where unwanted foods are available.** Your coworker has a bowl of candy on her desk? Meet the coworker in the cafeteria instead of her office. If you love pastry, don't drive past, park in front of, or keep the coupons for that store. Out of sight, out of mind.

- **Think of your cravings as something else.** Think of M&M's as marbles; pretzels become logs; marshmallows morph into clouds. Transform them into objects you can't or wouldn't want to eat.

- **Remember the consequences.** Those nachos are really hundreds of calories. Do you want those calories? Would you look as good in a bathing suit if that ice cream cone stuck out exactly where you know it will?

- **Limit snacks to those planned.** If you plan meals and snacks (during long stretches between some meals), you might be able to limit indulgence. So, look at your watch and anticipate the coming, scheduled eating event.

- **Avoid food commercials.** Food commercials on TV are timed to be viewed when the cravings can most influence sales. At least hit the mute button. Go put on your jammies[36] on instead of heading out the door or to the fridge to the find the food advertised.

- **Do something physical.** If you are busy, the cravings should bother you less. Walk. Stretch.

- **Head for the water fountain.** Thirst can mask as hunger. So, take a break with some water. Remember to avoid soda and beverages with artificial sweetener. On

---

36 The jammies trick only works if it is near your bedtime. Please don't tell your boss you're wearing jammies 'cause Ed said so!

your way back to what you were doing, focus on that activity and transition yourself back to what you were doing when the craving hit. What is the next step?

Know your food.

There are two sides of this coin. The first is to know about the foods you eat, and the second is to know more about food, in general.

Start paying attention to the labels on the foods you eat now. You can get a very interesting (disconcerting? disappointing? disgusting?) eye opener if you start reading the labels on the food you buy. High fructose corn syrup or other sugars, salt, preservatives, and hydrogenated[37] or trans fats, can lessen the nutritional value of your choices.

But the biggest surprise on the labels for me is the amount you should use to count as a serving. Did you know that a serving of

- Pizza is about a third of the *small* frozen pizza?
- Ice cream is about *half a cup*?
- The "individual-size" frozen potpie is just *half the pie*?
- Salad dressing is *only* two tablespoons?
- Condensed soup is *less than half* the cooked amount (after adding an equal measure of water)?

Finally, I've found it very helpful to learn more about foods. In particular, I read about foods you should eat and

---

37 Watch ingredient lists for "shortening" or the words "hydrogenated" or "partially hydrogenated." If found, make a different choice. These are often added to foods as preservatives, and they will be found in things such as French fries, snack foods, cookies, and some butter substitutes. Preservatives are designed to stick around, but they will also stick to the inside of your arteries. Not good.

foods you should avoid.[38] An easy way to do that is to read something every week. Health.com is an excellent source, as is ChooseMyPlate.gov.

Crys gets a daily email with recipes from two different organizations promoting healthier eating. She finds these helpful, particularly if we've had the "standard" tried-and-true recipe recently and need a change.

The same organization puts out a "food of the week" email and features that food on their website. Crys particularly likes having the information come to her rather than having to go find it on her own—if she thought to look for it.

These sources offer regular updates, more lists of five ways to improve this, ten things to avoid, and a video on cooking the other thing. A cornucopia of good information is out there. Dig in. Enjoy.

For You

The food journal shown in this chapter is available on the book website:

www.retireto.info/be-able/bookresources/

I've included two formats for ease of use. The first prints three to the page for trimming into the right size for a purse, gym bag or briefcase. The second format prints one to the page and is perfect for a three-ring notebook.

---

38 If you are using the food journal published on the Retire-To website for this book, it has a food tip or some kind of encouragement at the top of each page. Use these items as cues for more research. For example, one tip says to "Eat more MUFAs." If you don't already know what a MUFA is, use the log as an excuse to learn.

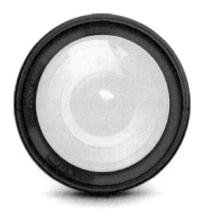

Conclusion

If you are like me and have found yourself overweight and out of shape, it may mean that at one time you weighed less, and you were likely in better shape. Most of us can reverse this transition. You found your way into the hole; you can find your way out of it too.

Exercising and eating well are not optional; they are the only ways to do what you want to do. Keep in mind four things:

> **Start**—Time waits for no man (or woman)!
>
> **Keep at it**—You are paid only if you show up for work!
>
> **Pay attention**—Convenience has consequences; eat well!
>
> **Don't give up**—Slow and steady wins the race! Getting to where you are now took time; getting to where you *want* to be will also take time—and persistence.

Don't assume how you feel now is the best you can be and you'll just decline as you age. With these steps, you can improve and maintain much longer.

But all things we've outlined in this book are just techniques. Techniques can be lost without the big picture. Who you are and how you want to be known and remembered are at stake here. Do you want to be the one who "languished until she died" or the one who "celebrated Thanksgiving with her family the night before she fell asleep and did not wake"?

> *Don't assume how you feel now is the best you can be. You can improve.*

Robert B. Parker's hero Spencer has always impressed me. Spencer once had a crisis of character when he faced recovery from a near-fatal bullet wound. He anguished over the consequences and the seemingly endless road to recovery. He asked his life-mate whether he would continue to be the toughest guy on the block. She told him something that's influenced me. She said that Spencer might not always be the strongest guy on the block, but he would always be the toughest!

She understood character. She understood that strength is a matter of biology but that being tough is a matter of character. But her truth rested in her conviction that character trumps ability—every time.

As we age, our bodies decline. Our character, on the other hand, can develop. When I talk about exercising, paying attention to nutrition, and embracing wellness, I'm not just talking about being better physically. I'm talking about development of a person—of you—a person with the conviction to relish life and willingness to reach for it. Cherish yourself, and push past any obstacles.

You need to stay in shape. But "staying in shape" means more than just exercising and eating well. It is an attitude.

It is a commitment. It represents determination, but not the grim determination it takes just to get through a difficult job. It is not about your force of will, but about the force of self that no longer has a need for excess weight and wants to exercise because it feels good. It is about discovering you and developing your character based on choice.[39]

What kind of person will you be? How will you be remembered? Isn't it odd that despite age, this question always stands before us? It is what life is about after all—a continual discovery of who you are.

I follow these four guidelines not just because I've achieved more than I ever imagined I could. I follow them because I want to be known as someone who pays attention, gets started, is not discouraged (for long), and keeps going. I won't last forever, but I want to leave at the top of my game regardless of how much I can still do physically.

Goodness knows, if I can achieve results, so can you. Have at it! I know you can do it. You can be able for the rest of your life. You can be a better you!

---

39 See www.consciousweightloss.com, created by Kathrine Brown, developer of the process, "Conscious Weight Loss: Bigger Life. Smaller Body."

Appendix

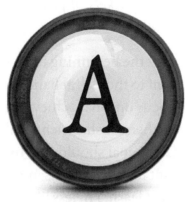

More on SMART Goals

SMART goal components

Start with **Specific** objectives. "I will make friends" is a laudable objective, but not a specific one. "I will meet Mike" is specific.

The specific objective in a SMART goal has to be **Measurable**. Putting a measurement to an objective helps you avoid vague or too-broad goals you cannot attain. If you can measure key elements, the goal is much more likely to be specific.

On the other hand, "I will make 5,000 cookies" is specific and measurable, but nearly unattainable. You can overdo. Watch that the goals you write are **Attainable**.

Relevant is also important. You have to pick actions that will make sense in context.

I will review three packets of pictures from my mother's ancient family collection this week.

This example shows the beginning of an excellent SMART goal. But it is irrelevant to the task at hand. Your SMART goals must maintain the focus on what achievements you envision. Writing those why or benefit statements will be helpful.

Finally, your SMART goal should be **<u>T</u>ime-bound**. Setting deadlines is important for two reasons: motivation and focus. If I know I'm on a short leash, I'm less likely to wander around chasing the wrong thing.

SMART goal examples

The following lists each start with an important step toward getting healthier. Under each heading are SMART goals that are examples of how to go about meeting the overall objective. Each example includes the SMART elements—**S**pecific, **M**easurable, **A**ttainable, **R**elevant, **T**ime-bound.[40]

#1 Establish a benchmark.

- This week, I will visit bluezones.com and measure my current habits on the "Vitality Compass," a two-minute tool.
- While at the gym tomorrow, I'll check the possibility of getting a fitness assessment from a personal trainer. I want a personalized program for improvement so I can track my efforts and progress.

---

40 This list was generated from participant input at the New 3Rs of Retirement workshops my wife, Crys, and I have conducted in the Nashville area.

#2 Learn, learn, learn.

- Maybe the library has subscriptions to *Prevention* or *Health* magazines. I'll look when I go to the library tomorrow. I'd like to see what they are like before ordering a subscription for myself.
- By next Friday, I'll search the Internet for… (whatever interests you—local bicycling clubs, wellness classes, new walking shoes, and so on).

#3 Try some new dishes.

- We're going out to celebrate a birthday tomorrow night; I'll find and order a meal (the vegetarian option?) that will get more plant-based food into my diet.
- By Tuesday, I'll call my friend Jim (Jack, Brendon, whomever) and invite him to dinner. I'll cook a special vegetable.
- Time to explore some new recipes. By next Friday, I'll look for a copy of *Cooking Light* magazine. A subscription might be in order so I can get regular advice for a while.
- The hospital (the grocery store, community college, church, and so on) offers a "healthy" cooking class. By next Tuesday, I'll register for a class. I would like to practice making a recommended dish.
- By next Monday, I will cook one new dinner item. I intend to repeat the practice weekly.

#4 Get moving.

- There are several greenways nearby. I'll walk one by next Tuesday.

- The Silver Sneakers program is good, I'm told. By Saturday, I'll look that up on the web and see what the local options are.

- We bought a Wii for the grandkids. I wonder whether there is a Wii activity that suits me, perhaps the Wii Fit balance board. Tomorrow I'll start bowling on my Wii and, by next Friday, check other games.

- I think the dog needs to walk more often and farther. We'll go around our usual route twice tonight and keep that up for a week.

- I sit too much at the computer. I need to move in place more. I saw a video about getting up and doing stretches hourly. I'm going to look up that video tonight.

#5 Get a buddy.

- My wife and I can figure out things to do together to be more active at the desk. Let's talk about it at dinner tonight.

- Clare mentioned she had a bike. I'll call her by tomorrow to see if we can set a time to ride together.

Appendix

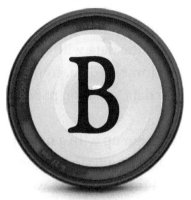

Personal Health Records

Why keep a Personal Health Record (PHR)

The need for you to maintain a personal record of your medical history, conditions, and overall health is based on one simple notion—doctors are not the source of your medical records they once were.

Growing up in small-town Ohio, I had a physician who was the only source of medical information about me—and probably several hundred others in the county. Not true anymore. Today you probably have a primary-care physician (PCP), but unless you are conscientious about asking specialists, eye doctors, dentists, and clinics to send details to that physician, you simply can't rely on your PCP to have all that information.

Consider, too, that our care in general these days is based on much more information than years ago, which means that even if you could store the data with one caregiver, it may be difficult, given the volume of data, to find a particular detail or to spot trends. The data, often on paper, is voluminous and not easily searched.

It's even difficult to sign up with a new specialist. He or she wants answers to reams of questions. Sometimes, the details are "lost in the mist of time." In other words, that stuff is hard to remember.

You need to keep track—in writing. And you may want to use a computer to help you. Your personal records might be the only complete data available. Besides, if you keep track of the details, you get more involved in your care.

Many computer programs are available to help track personal medical data. When you start to evaluate which would work for you, keep in mind four goals.

The system should

- **Record and track the data** that you need and that captures your interest. You will not enter data into a computer unless you expect to achieve some result. So, start by asking what data you want and need.
- **Help spot trends.** Is my blood pressure getting to where it needs to be? Is my cholesterol level headed in the right direction?
- **Point out anomalies.** Sudden weight gain or loss may point to other problems.
- **Facilitate data transport.** Getting the data to the next doctor in line is important. Doctors come and go. Your health records do not. You can avoid having to remember the details with every new care provider who requires them.

I began my review of available systems with the Medicare record-keeping system.[41] The data collected seems extensive, particularly about personal medical history: conditions, allergies, implants, immunizations, vital statistics, and lab and test results.

Healthcare providers add some data from the Medicare system automatically. However, this only works to the users' advantage if providers make claims directly to Medicare. Because I'm a member of an Advantage plan, the information on this site is spotty for me (the point of an Advantage plan is that Medicare doesn't have to track what you do).

MyMedicare.gov has a chat feature that allows you to access help readily.

More PHR information

You can get more information about personal health records at the following websites:

Medline Plus[42] is a service of the US National Library of Medicine National Institutes of Health that gives overview information about such systems. This site is a wealth of information about all kinds of health topics. Use the links to explore different questions.

MyPHR,[43] sponsored by the American Health Information Management Association, seems more extensive. It offers a form you can print and complete to start your record keeping. In addition, it lists dozens of available computer program options.

---

41 At Medicare.gov, create an account and navigate to the page called MyMedicare. When you return to the website, you can go directly to MyMedicare.gov and log on.

42 http://www.nlm.nih.gov

43 http://www.myphr.com

PHR Examples

I'm also listing two software systems among the dozens out there. The Microsoft product is unique in its collaborative work with many, many vendors. (Remember, you are interested in only the collaborations you need.)

myMediConnect [44] offers service as well as data storage; for a fee, they will dig out the information for you. myMediConnect is one example of the many fee-based portals available. I mention it to illustrate two other services that might interest you. First, for a per-doctor fee, this company will upload and store medical records from your physicians. Your doctors will not release this information without your consent, so myMediConnect offers a HIPPA release form.

Microsoft HealthVault [45] has a wealth of partners to track your medical details. For example, if you work with CVS or Walgreens pharmacies (or others), this software can upload your prescription history as well as future details. If you read the information in Chapter 3 about the Fitbit device I carry, you'll be interested to know that the Fitbit will supply information directly to HealthVault so you can track activity history in one place. HealthVault also partners with companies that make

    Heart rate monitors
    Blood pressure monitors
    Peak flow meters
    Glucometers

HealthVault advertises a service that claims to eliminate the "clipboard" by uploading data to the doctor's office directly.

---

44 https://www.mymediconnect.net
45 https://www.healthvault.com

Similar to Microsoft, myMediConnect securely stores your data in the Cloud so you can retrieve it wherever you are (including your doctor's office). When you visit a new doctor, you can access details to complete the form.

One other benefit: Both Microsoft HealthVault and myMediConnect offer smartphone or tablet access to your data. You can print your records to carry to the doctor's office, or you can just carry your phone.

Here is a list of the data important for your record keeping. Various systems record some of these details; others pick a different set. Buyer, beware! Decide the details you need to track before selecting a software product.

Personal and Basic Health Information
>   Name, address, gender, phone number, email address, date of birth,
>   Medicare effective dates, height, weight, blood type

Healthcare Providers

Allergies
>   Environmental and those related to food and medications

Medical Conditions

Pharmacies

Medications
>   Over-the-counter
>   Prescription

Family Medical History

Implanted Devices

Vital Statistics
>   Blood pressure
>   Temperature
>   Glucose level

Preventive Services
Labs and Tests
Immunizations
Plans and Coverage
Emergency Contacts
        Primary and Alternative
Uploaded documents
        Living will
        Medical directives

Other Books by Ed Zinkiewicz

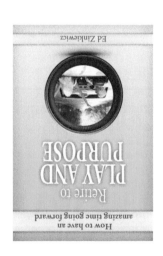

Retire to Play and Purpose
How to have an amazing time
going forward

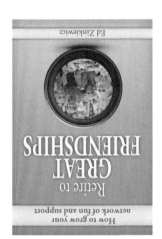

Retire to Great Friendships
How to grow your network of
fun and support

**Find more details about these
and other resources at**

Retire-To.com